D0793080

The Spiritual Teachings of
YOGA

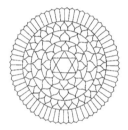

The Special Yoga Centre
The Tay Building
2a Wrentham Avenue
London NW10 3HA

Tel: +44 208 968 1900
www.specialyoga.org.uk

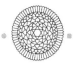

Also by Mark Forstater

The Spiritual Teachings of Marcus Aurelius

The Spiritual Teachings of the Tao

The Spiritual Teachings of Seneca
(also by Victoria Radin)

The Living Wisdom of Socrates

Visit The Special Yoga Centre website at:
www.specialyoga.org.uk

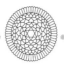

The Spiritual Teachings of
YOGA

Jo Manuel and
Mark Forstater

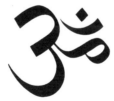

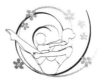

The Special Yoga Centre

To Cleo and Lily with all our love.
May your light always shine brightly.

Copyright © 2008 by Jo Manuel and Mark Forstater

Published in 2008 by Mark Forstater Productions Ltd.

The right of Mark Forstater and Jo Manuel to be identified as the Authors
of the Work has been asserted by them in accordance with the Copyright,
Designs and Patents Act 1988.

1 3 5 7 9 10 8 6 4 2

'Yoga-seal' reproduced from Flood, Gavin, *An Introduction to Hinduism*,
Cambridge University Press (1996).

A CIP catalogue record for this title is available
from the British Library

ISBN 978 0 9558885 1 9

Typeset in Photina by Palimpsest Book Production Limited,
Polmont, Stirlingshire

Printed and bound in Great Britain by
Athenaeum Press Ltd.

Mark Forstater Productions Ltd.
11 Keslake Road
London NW6 6DJ

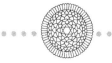

Contents

Acknowledgements

The authors would like to mention the following people for helping them in the creation of this book and audiotape.

Jo:
There are so many wonderful people I have met over the many years that I have practised yoga who have helped me to follow my path. It would take up pages and pages to list them all . . . but thanks to all of you. My special and heart-felt thanks to the many teachers that I have had the good fortune to be taught and inspired by, among whom are: Dharma, my first yoga teacher who in the 1980s had a love-ly little centre on West 4th Street in New York City and who to this day is one of the most centred and peaceful people I have ever met; Faustomaria; Mary Stewart; Catherine James, who lovingly encouraged me to train to teach; Helen Elliott; John Stirk, Peter Blackaby and Sophie Hoare who not only trained me to teach but gave me their words of wis-dom and inspired me with their deep love and knowledge of yoga; the late Vanda Scaravelli who has so inspired my prac-tice and teaching; Dominique Moorsom, Monica Voss and Anne Marie Zulkahari whose deep loving friendship, joy and fun is so much appreciated; Swami Satchidananda whose beautiful ashram I had the honour to live at while doing the Yoga for the Special Child course; and Sonia Sumar, who embodies light and love in her work with spe-cial children. And many thanks also to all my students: the adults, the children and the special needs children who have undoubtedly taught me as much, if not more, than I have taught them.

Writing this book was an honour and a learning curve; some days I didn't know that I would be able to complete it.

My thanks to those who helped encourage me on the way, particularly Liane Jones, Michele Cohen, Wendy Oberman, Anni Girling, Lisette Keats, Barbara Hezelgrave and Kate Stone for their friendship and encouragement, boosting my confidence when needed. I would like to give very special thanks to my wonderful brother Doug for always being there for me and without whom my life would not be the same.

Special thanks also to Mark for agreeing to write this book and then giving me the opportunity to write it with him. Delving into the depths of this wonderful and enlightening philosophy has changed my understanding of life, enhanced my yoga practice and brought me closer to God.

Mark:

To my editors, Rowena Webb at Hodder Mobius and Trena Keating at Plume, many thanks for continuing to support this series.

Thanks to Rupert Lancaster, editor of Hodder Audio, for your support and help on the audio version.

Much appreciation to my agent Liv Blumer for all her help and support in getting the series noticed internationally.

To Harry, Doug, Frank and Lucille for reading drafts and giving valuable suggestions.

To Joan Corlass for her lovely Sanskrit calligraphy.

To Harry and Irene who put me up and put up with me in the last throes of the introduction.

To Dominique Moorsom for her wonderful instruction at Le Montizon and to Dawn for her fine cooking.

I would like to express my appreciation to the many dedicated Indian and yoga scholars, both East and West, whose works I have read with great interest and used as the foundation for my conclusions and beliefs. Without their pioneering work, this book could not have been written.

And finally to Jo, my yoga teacher, mentor, editor and cowriter, who first suggested doing this book, and whose work on the yoga texts will make these available and accessible to many people. Writing this book has enabled me to add the theoretical part of yoga to my existing practice, to the improvement of both. More importantly, writing with you has brought us closer together, and I hope that we can both grow from this experience.

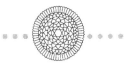

Lead us from the unreal to the real.
Lead us from darkness to light.
Lead us from the fear of death
to knowledge of immortality.
BRIHADARANYAKA UPANISHAD

PART ONE

Yoga is a Living Philosophy

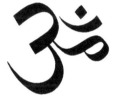

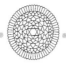

Preface

Yoga is India's greatest gift to the world.
KRISHNAMACHARYA

We think we 'do' yoga, but the Indian term 'yoga' encompasses much more than the health and fitness regime that is largely practised in the West.

Originally developed in India nearly 6,000 years ago as a method of integrating the entire person and of freeing the spirit, yoga is sometimes seen today as another form of aerobics, a stress reducer or a means to a flatter tummy. It's true that yoga makes our bodies stronger, more agile and flexible, and our minds more relaxed, but the ultimate aim of yoga practice is to go beyond these limited results and to unite all aspects of the person: mind, body, heart and spirit. It is in this sense that it can be called a spiritual practice.

The ancient teachers considered yoga to be a science, since its aim is to help us to gain knowledge – not the external knowledge of facts, figures and intellectual learning, but the deepest and most intimate interior knowledge we can have, that of our true inner selves. And this knowledge is not narcissistic or solipsistic, because one of the goals of yoga is to make us feel more at one with ourselves, whilst at the same time improving our important and intimate relationships with the world. Yoga is often called the science of Self-realization, because its end result is a realization of just who we are, not limiting that knowledge to our surface personality, or the ego-led persona that we project out into the world, but discovering the real person, the Self hidden deep inside, which yoga declares to be Spirit itself.

There is a wealth of living philosophy behind yoga that,

once understood and combined with practice, can make our yoga training deeper, stronger and more satisfying. With this knowledge we are able to bring yoga into all aspects of our daily lives and use it to extend, deepen and enhance our approach to life.

Part One of this book (by Mark Forstater) accessibly explains and clarifies the history and ideas that underpin yoga practice, bringing in fresh analogies and examples that illuminate both theory and practice. Part Two (by yoga teacher and therapist Jo Manuel) presents the key spiritual texts that relate to yoga theory in a clear and poetic style. These texts are the major *Upanishads*, the *Bhagavad Gita*, and the *Yoga Sutras* of Patanjali, which date from the sixth century BCE to the second century CE.

Someone once wrote that yoga would eventually unite East and West. With the explosion of interest in yoga today, this prospect may not be that far off. But it's important that the yoga that might unite us in this new century operates on a spiritual as well as on a physical level. It is the authors' hope that this book will show people how to make these spiritual connections work and in its own way aid in making this important unity a reality.

We began writing this book during a dark time, a time that the Hindus call the Kali Yuga, the Age of Iron, which they describe as a long period of decline and degeneration. This preface was in its earliest stages when the devastating terrorist attack on the Pentagon and the World Trade Center, an event now known as 9/11, took place.

The 9/11 atrocity starkly revealed to us two distinct aspects of human experience: tragedy and courage, evil and good, ugliness and beauty, the highest ideals and the lowest venality. The pain and suffering of the innocents caught in the burning buildings brought forth waves of compassion from the countless millions who witnessed the tragedy on television. At the same time, the untold acts of mercy, heroism and bravery exhibited by police officers, fire-fighters and ordinary civilians, who gave selflessly of themselves without a thought to their own safety, filled us all with admiration.

What can we learn from this event? How can we make sense of something that seems so senseless? Were the suffering and pain of the dead and injured without meaning? What lessons can be learned from the sorrow and grief of those left behind, who must now try, for the rest of their lives, to make sense of what seems utterly senseless, the wanton destruction of human life for a religious or political cause.

We need to see 9/11 as a catalyst, an event that acted, and will act in future, as an agent for transformation and change. This transformation is from a largely materialistic society, dominated by loneliness, greed, competition and violence, to one where spirituality and its higher values of sharing, compassion and community will take precedence.

Why do I think this will happen? First, the impressive acts of selfless courage on 9/11 demonstrated that even in the midst of the most evil events, there is still the possibility to display the best of human qualities, our tremendous capacity for good. Second, the world was brought together to witness this awful tragedy, and the universal feelings of compassion and solidarity that were expressed gave a renewed impetus to spiritual feelings all over the globe. In their shock and confusion, people turned to one another, and to prayer; places of worship were packed.

Experience and history tell us that, however awful any single event may appear, there will always be a response to it, a reaction from it, or a consequence of it, that will eventually produce good. Yoga teaching says that all events are really equal, and that our response to them should be even and steady. In yoga we train ourselves to see the world as a balanced equality, in which the opposites, as in Yin – Yang theory, always find an equilibrium. This is also the lesson of the Law of Karma, that says that all actions become reactions, and causes become effects *ad infinitum*, since our world is a web made of an infinite and endless series of causes and effects. Difficult as it may be to learn to see the world in this way, it does lead to an extremely positive outlook on life, one that can find true contentment in human existence.

More than ever, what we need is a transformation of attitude that can help us adapt to the many unwelcome changes facing us in this dark and dangerous new century and to the uncertainties and fears that accompany our new political situation. We need to find a new vision, a new way of looking at the world and ourselves, to discover a different and better way to act towards our fellow human beings and to protect the damaged earth we live and depend upon. Unless we can find this new vision and discover a way to renew ourselves, our Western way of life may go into the dustbin of history with all the other ancient societies that failed to adapt to radical change.

In this new century that has begun with such universal fear and uncertainty, we believe that yoga can provide us with the means to find this new vision and to discover a calm and stable centre that will help us survive this dangerous and insecure time. From this place of inner peace, we can find a compassion that will radiate outwards to other people, to animals and to the earth itself. It is only from the serenity of this inner peace that a true outer peace and sense of security can be established.

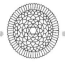

I

A View from Above

When I was a kid, my parents took me to the top of the Empire State Building in New York, then the tallest man-made structure in the world. From its unbelievably high and windy observation platform I looked down on the busy streets below, watching people as small as insects scurrying through the square stone canyons of Manhattan. As I gazed straight down from the immense height of the eighty-sixth floor, everyone at street level looked so minuscule that they had lost their normal identity, colours and individuality.

Down below everything was so tiny that individual movements were difficult to focus on and I became aware only of mass actions. The people moving on the sidewalk were no longer people but resembled conglomerations of anonymous mobile black dots, moving with some kind of organized, almost mechanized, purpose, like figures from an early video game. From this height there seemed to be little difference between a person and a car, since both moved *en masse*, and whether this movement was conscious or mechanical could not be determined. It was like watching cells under a microscope, aware of some kind of intelligent activity, but an intelligence alien to your own.

A few years later, I had a similar experience watching an anthill on scrubland. Looking again from above, I saw that the actions of the ants were also collective rather than individual as they moved to and from the nest in their hundreds, in long files, those arriving carrying bits of leaves or crumbs incredibly large for their delicate and intricate bodies. They all followed the same paths, sometimes wandering off but always curving back to join the long supply lines stretching out from their home to the weedy and litter-filled ground.

Seeing such purposeful activity, it seemed odd not to credit the ants with consciousness. Certainly keen intelligence seemed to be on display in such a highly controlled organization. All the ants seemed busy, all had jobs to do, none slacked off or stood around bickering. Their activity was as purposeful as that of the streets of Manhattan. Apparently an ant's intelligence is completely tied up with its instinct, so that the highly structured ant societies with their diversity of fixed jobs never vary. As far as we can tell, no ant ever becomes self-reflective enough to question his or her role in life, to investigate some other behaviour, or even take a day off work.

Thinking back to my elevated view in New York, and considering the anonymous dots of people also flowing purposefully along, I wondered how much our own actions might also be due to instinct tied to intelligence. If we look carefully at what we do and how we live our lives, we find ourselves wondering how much genuine thought we actually take over our actions, or do we in truth act largely through habit, memory and conditioned responses, almost like Pavlov's dogs? What is it that makes us so different from ants?

Although to an extent we're creatures of instinct and fall easily into habit, we have a more open-ended, adaptable and creative intelligence than ants, one capable of being developed to a very high degree, that has enabled us, among many other things, to paint pictures, write songs and discover the physical laws that govern the universe. We are able to employ symbols, to think abstractly, and to consider the nature of our own consciousness. The seven wonders of the world cannot compare with just this one wonder – that of the human spirit, our most precious asset.

The people I looked at in the streets below seemed so insignificant, completely bereft of individuality. Yet what we consider the most important part of ourselves *is* our individuality, the quality of being a person, a significant and special creature whose existence makes a difference in the totality of the universe.

It is unlikely that an ant would ever ask the four fundamental questions of Tantra Yoga:

Who am I?
Where have I come from?
Where am I going?
Why am I here?

These questions go to the heart of what it means to be human. They represent some of the most profound mysteries of life, which most of us at some time feel compelled to consider. This curiosity becomes a search for spiritual knowledge, an understanding that cannot be discovered by examining only the outside. It is an inner quest, one that we pursue naturally when very young, before we become conditioned by our parents, teachers and increasingly the media to accept their version of reality. This curiosity emerges again later in life, when with increasing age we reflect on ourselves and our place in the world.

We are all unique, we are all individual and special. Yet our lives are not at all equal. We are happy or suffer in different ways. What matters to most of us is primarily our own individual happiness. But in pursuing that happiness we often discover paradoxically that it recedes from our grasp, and instead of happiness increasing it is our unhappiness that grows. That unhappiness brings with it the four horsemen of our personal apocalypse: frustration, anger, anguish and despair.

When this happens we feel confused and lost, and if we are determined enough we become searchers, seekers after a new truth, one which we hope can offer us some kind of salvation and hope. Asking these fundamental questions of existence, we seek out people, ideas or movements that claim to have a handle on the truth, hoping that one of them will give us an answer, or at least show us the path along which answers can be found.

Many paths are offered today, but one that has become immensely popular over the past thirty years is yoga, which is also the oldest spiritual path we know of. For over 5,000 years the teachings of yoga have provided a way for those who seek a deep meaning in life, a connection with a power greater than themselves, and whose goal is the liberation of their spirit.

As individuals we sometimes find it hard to see any purpose in our lives, and a life without purpose or meaning feels barren and empty, devoid of taste and pleasure. We don't want to be collective automatons like ants, which is where our technology seems to be herding us, but we appear to lack the means to fight against these developments. We are in danger of losing contact with our souls, and without that link we can't seem to find the purpose and meaning of existence.

Can we find a way to get it back? Can we discover in ourselves a rich and vibrant soul, a creative spirit that initiates and receives love, comfort and joy out of our ordinary mundane existence? Can we in fact transform our seemingly mundane lives into a form of the sacred?

This book explores these ideas, and shows how yoga was designed to establish a fully developed, fully creative, fully functioning human being, a man or woman able to live life to the full, with a strong, flexible body and a clear, active mind, as well as vibrant emotions that enable one to share life with others in loving, supportive relationships.

2

The Aim of Yoga

M ost books on yoga begin with a definition of the word 'yoga' and I'm not about to break with hallowed tradition. Yoga, we are told, is a Sanskrit term that comes from the root *yuj*, meaning to join, connect, unite and so on, and is related to the English word 'yoke', meaning to restrain or harness. Now, the word yoke used to be on everyone's tongue in the pre-automobile age, when we used oxen or horses to plough our fields and to transport ourselves and our goods. The yoke went over the horses' necks and connected them to the plough or wagon, thereby harnessing their power to pull the vehicle.

The image of horses pulling chariots is a familiar one in Indian scriptures, and as early as the sixth century BCE the Hindu rishis, or sages, used this image of horse and chariot in a symbolic way to represent the nature of the human mind, its wayward impulses and desires. The following passage is from the *Katha Upanishad*, a speculative philosophical text:

> *Look on the Eternal Spirit as the ruler of a chariot, and the body as the chariot itself; reason is the driver and the mind the reins it holds; the horses are the senses, while selfish desires are the roads they travel on.*
>
> *The sages say that when we confuse the Eternal Spirit with the body, mind and senses, we suffer pain and enjoy pleasure,*

but have no real joy. When a person lacks steadiness and is unable to control his mind, his senses are like wild horses. But the mind, like horses, can be trained.

In terms of contemporary yoga practice, what is it that we are harnessing? Unlike horsepower, we are not just harnessing the power of our bodies, but rather training the power of our minds. The purpose of yoga, as defined in the *Yoga Sutras*, the most ancient (fourth- to third-century BCE) text of yoga philosophy, is to stop the wandering and craving mind and return it to a serene and calm state. The *Yoga Sutras* don't instruct on how to get into physical postures, as we might expect, but instead explain how the mind works, and how to train it. Paradoxically, the power of the mind is unleashed not by allowing it to be increasingly active, but by encouraging it to become centred and stilled. As the *Yoga Sutra* says,

Yoga means to control and still the swirling currents of thoughts in the mind. If you can control the thoughts that arise, and still them completely, you are able to observe the world clearly and directly without the distortions of the ego. The ability to discipline the chattering mind is what takes us to the state of yoga.
When the turbulence stops and the lake of the mind becomes clear and still, our true essence, our Self, is reflected. Then the Self can abide in its own true nature. This is the goal, this is what we want to attain.

Yoga encourages us to let go of unnecessary desires, thereby learning to quieten and concentrate the mind, increasing our ability to direct it in ways that will give us greater control over our senses and our minds, thoughts and feelings, desires and impulses. This control is not repressive and strict, but represents a more balanced and harmonious approach to life, one that can restore in us a sense of joy.

A second meaning of the word yoga is to unite, and it is here that we come across many different interpretations of what it is that is being united. The essence of these interpretations is that yoga enables us to unite our inner Self with a higher, more universal Spirit or power, whether we call this power God, Allah, YHWH, Brahman, the Absolute, the Eternal, the Great Spirit, Tao, Buddha, Nature and so on. The yogis believe that all these names refer to the same source, a cosmic energy or power that all religions have discovered. As Swami Satchidananda says, repeating an ancient yogic saying:

There is one truth.
There are many paths.

Yoga, by uniting our individual Self with this higher truth, can give us a more expansive and extended view of life. Yoga also enables us to unite our complete being, so that body, breath, mind, spirit and heart become integrated as one and we no longer feel cut off, separated and isolated from each other and from the rest of creation. We understand in a visceral way (not merely intellectually) that we are not isolated creatures in a cold and alien universe, but are connected in a great web of being with everything that exists. I don't know if the novelist E. M. Forster ever practised yoga, but he understood the need for it when he told us, 'Only connect.' If we can acquire such a state of cosmic connectedness we are in a position to fulfil our own unique and individual potential.

Life is a journey, and if we're lucky, we are able to find a spiritual path to follow, a living philosophy or way of life that guides us safely through the difficulties and dangers of that journey. Yoga is just such a spiritual path that can take us on a journey from wherever we start, perhaps as limited and contracted people, into a more expanded and inclusive person. So the word yoga also means to go on a journey of discovery from here to beyond.

Yoga also means perfect action, because once we have achieved a union of our deepest spiritual Self with the universe, having lost or diminished many of our unnecessary desires and selfish ego limitations, we suddenly find ourselves acting spontaneously and correctly in all life's situations. Once all our parts have become integrated and work together properly, we respond naturally and holistically to events. By changing how we respond to events, yoga can have a direct and positive influence on our lives. It is a practical vision leading to practical results.

When the West first became aware of yoga, it was associated with wiry Indian men in loincloths who contorted their bodies into pretzel shapes in order to gain supernatural powers. These magical powers included the ability to read minds, to be in two places at once, to see into the future and so on. A famous experiment took place early in the nineteenth century in India in an attempt to prove that these powers were real and not illusory. A famous saddhu (holy man) named Haridas allowed himself to be buried alive by the Maharaja of Lahore. Haridas had his beard shaved and laid himself in a chest sealed with the Maharaja's royal seal. The chest was then buried in earth and sown with barley seed. The burial area was enclosed by a wall and guarded day and night by armed soldiers.

Four months later, when Haridas was exhumed, barley was growing on the earth. When the saddhu was taken out of the chest, his facial hair had not grown at all and he was still alive. Yoga had given him so much control over his bodily processes that he was able to put himself into a state of suspended animation, a kind of hibernation.

Most people in the West don't practise yoga to acquire

special powers like these, but yoga is popularly seen as a form of physical exercise that children, adults and the aged can do to gain fitness or to reduce stress. This emphasis on the physical side of yoga limits the amount of spiritual benefits that can accrue, but there is no doubt that even limited yoga training increases health and well-being, as B.K.S Iyengar, who has been one of the most influential teachers of Hatha Yoga in the West, emphasizes:

Physical health is important for mental development, as normally the mind functions through the nervous system. When the body is sick or the nervous system affected, the mind becomes restless or dull and inert and concentration or meditation become impossible.

Yoga was conceived by the ancient Indian rishis as a practical method for the complete physical, mental and spiritual transformation of the individual. We are often told, 'To change your life you only need to change your mind. If you change your mind, the way you see the world, you and your world will automatically change.' As the Buddha said,

All that we are is the result of what we have thought. We are made of our thoughts.

I believe this is true, but I also know that it is not only very difficult to change the way you see the world, but even harder to maintain a new vision, and not backslide into old and habitual conditioning, losing the very gains you have made.

Yoga philosophy explains why it is so difficult to effect this change of mind. To the yogis the mind was virtually the sixth sense, in that it was similar in physical substance and function to the other five senses, which report to it. We have a saying, 'Mind over matter', but the yogis wouldn't agree with this idea. To them, mind is not separate from matter but partakes of matter, even if it is a finer and more subtle manifestation of it. For the yogis, mind is not spirit, and one of the reasons why it is so difficult to alter the mind in any semi-permanent way is that it is so intimately tied up with the body, the senses and their objects of desire. The *Katha Upanishad* says:

Beyond the senses are the objects of desire,
beyond the objects of desire is the mind,
beyond the mind is the intellect,
beyond the intellect is our true nature
and our true Self.

To change the mind, you also need to alter the body, which is why yoga has a body–mind co-ordinated approach to the problem.

By persevering with a yoga practice of postures, breathing and meditation, there is a steady alteration of the physical habits of the body, and this in itself alters the mind, through the mind–body connection. The regular practice of asanas (postures) makes you more aware of your body, how you use it and how your breath functions, and this understanding allows you to alter the way you hold yourself, move and breathe. These changes will naturally, according to yoga philosophy, alter the way you use your mind.

Your mind can behave as a good friend, but also as your enemy. The uncontrolled mind acts as your enemy.

As you gain control of your mind with the help of your higher Self, you are a friend of your higher Self, and your mind and ego become your friends. When your mind is disciplined and your soul is at peace, so you are in peace and remain unaffected by heat or cold, pleasure or pain, praise or blame.

Yoga's influence in the East for nearly 6,000 years is due to the fact that it is a completely worked out and fully tested system of process for change. This change works on the entire person and has an effect on the physical body, the mind, the emotions and the spirit. The danger of backsliding was known to the ancient yogis and sages who worked out this system, and they incorporated this problem into it. I believe that anyone who wants to effect change in themselves will find that yoga has the potential for a total transformation of their person. Since an open body leads to an open heart, yoga starts with a renewal of the body and leads to a rejuvenation of the Spirit.

Of course, not everyone wants to transform themselves completely, but most people would quite like to improve their health, lose some weight, or put some calm and contentment into stressed lives. To make such changes requires that we alter old, negative habits into new, healthier ones. To alter old conditioning, such as poor diet, smoking, or drug habits, or damaging personal and sexual attitudes, can only be accomplished through a transformation of the mind. Since yoga specifically targets the mind, with the aim of increasing control over it, yoga practice can help us effect these character changes without having to alter our religion, become vegetarian, give up sex or completely change our way of life.

There is no need to believe in yoga philosophy to get real benefit from yoga practice. The power of asanas, pranayama (breath control), and meditation, the three main aspects of yoga practice in the West, are more than sufficient to have a very positive effect on our entire being. As the *Amritabindu Upanishad* states,

The mind can be both pure and impure. Driven by the senses it becomes impure, but with the senses under control the mind can become pure. It is the mind that frees us or enslaves us. When we are driven by the senses we become bound; if we

seek freedom we must master our senses. When the mind is detached from the senses we reach the height of awareness. Mastery of the mind leads to wisdom.

A. G. Mohan, in his excellent book *Yoga for Body, Breath and Mind*, makes the point that yoga is both a process, a means to an end, and the end itself, the result of that process. The process of yoga is the practice that is most obvious in the asanas or postures that our body moves into and holds. Since this is so visible, it's what most people think of when they hear the word yoga.

I first started practising Hatha Yoga, which is the yoga that we mainly do in the West, about ten years ago, at the suggestion of my wife Jo, who had been a serious yoga student for many years. She was pregnant at the time, and as I was going to be a father again (at fifty), she thought it prudent that I get my body in shape to be able to take on the new tasks of lifting and carrying our new bundle of joy.

I attended a couple of Jo's classes at a yoga centre and soon realized just how unfit and inflexible my body was. I was unable to touch the floor when bending over because my spine was quite rigid – when I sat on the floor, legs outstretched, I could barely bend forward. My shoulders and neck were very tense, and I held still more tension in my belly and diaphragm. I had tight hamstring (upper-leg) muscles, cramped calf muscles and tense upper-arm muscles. My pelvis was virtually immobile. In short, my body was a mess.

In the classes, I urged my body to move into the positions that everyone else seemed just to float into, but I was unable to match their easy and practised postures. It was clear that my first task would be slowly to undo long-standing tensions that I had accumulated through lack of physical exercise and by holding in my body the accumulated stresses of negative emotions and thoughts. In the end, this process of undoing took quite a number of years, is still taking place, and as Jo often reminds me, will never come to an end, as there is always more to undo!

The yoga asanas or postures work primarily on the muscles, since these are virtually the only parts of the body over which we have conscious control. We can make the muscles move as we like, subject only to our physical limitations, which in my case were many. So a well-structured yoga practice is designed to move our body, in co-ordination with the breath, into a variety of positions that will undo the body by stretching, exercising and strengthening all our muscles. Allowing the breath to soften the muscles lets us release them, and this in turn creates space in the spine and in the joints, allowing us to breathe into them. This freeing of muscles and skeletal connections rids the entire body of tension and permits the body's natural intelligence to function. Since the spine protects the central nervous system, any improvement in the spine's flexibility immediately improves the working of the nervous system itself.

In those first classes my body showed little sign of intelligence – it was more like the dunce of the class. As I moved into the asanas I became aware of a sharp, burning sensation in the muscles that I was working, as they were being stretched beyond their comfort zone. According to the *Yoga Sutras*, the positions we take should be easy and comfortable, not difficult and painful, and the rule 'No pain, no gain' is not really part of yoga. However 'No burn, no earn' reflects the fact that unless we reach our bodies' limitations we are not able to go beyond them.

When we start yoga, even when we have trained for a while, there will always be positions that are uncomfortable. But a qualified and experienced teacher will show us how to breathe ourselves safely into these positions and so feel a gradual letting go of tense muscles. Learning how to work with the breath, using its natural healing and liberating qualities, is one of yoga's most important and pleasant lessons. Through the skilful use of the breath we know that progress is being made without harm. But if we force ourselves into positions that are painful and try to maintain them on the basis that the pain is necessary, we will be working against ourselves and may cause injury.

At the end of these first yoga sessions, my body felt calm and smooth, with a sense of fluidity, of starting to move lightly and composedly. My body felt as though it was beginning to cohere again, to integrate like a well-oiled machine: fluid in motion, co-ordinated and smooth.

After a couple of years I stopped yoga to learn Tai Chi, and then returned once more, as a beginner, to yoga training. Over the last few years, little by little, my tight muscles are slowly giving way and the tense joints of my body are loosening, so that I am able to move much more freely than before. My spine in particular has lost much of its rigidity and I have regained an agility and energy that I thought were lost forever. Connected once more to my body, I found its inner rhythm through the use of movement and breath. Suddenly, I enjoyed dancing again.

The feeling I had is corroborated by Iyengar:

The right method of doing asanas brings lightness and an exhilarating feeling in the body and the mind and a feeling of oneness.

The practice of asanas is very effective on the body's muscles and nerves, but on its own cannot undo those long-standing physical and mental obstructions that stop us from acting and living freely. These blockages, both mental and physical, are caused by the mind, not by the body. The process of yoga that A. G. Mohan wrote about is not an exclusively external process that works with the body but an internal one that works with the breath and the mind.

This internal process works from the outside in, from the gross or heavy to the subtle. So although we begin our yoga practice working with the body (in co-ordination with the breath), which is the gross part of our nature, we then focus more exclusively on the breath, which is finer, and end up in a state of meditation in which we work directly with the mind, which is finer and more subtle still. This gradual focusing inwards eventually leads to a state of samadhi, when all thoughts are stilled, the mind quietens, the senses withdraw from the busy noisy outside world and we find ourselves absorbed in a blissful and peaceful awareness of primal consciousness.

This state of translucency and peace is called liberation and goes by the Sanskrit word *moksha*. Although there are many types of yoga – Hatha Yoga, Karma Yoga, Bhakti Yoga, Mantra Yoga, Kriya Yoga, Raja Yoga, Laya Yoga, and others – they all have as their ultimate aim liberation, the freeing of our inner Self or Spirit from a false illusion created by the mind.

What does liberation feel like? Never having fully experienced it, I can't tell you, and those who have say that it can't be put into words. Like describing the smell of a flower or the taste of honey, the limitations of words and concepts fail to come close to conveying living experience. All we can do if we want to find out is to take up yoga practice ourselves, so that we can directly understand what this state of consciousness feels like. Subtle and mysterious experiences are so entirely subjective that they cannot be conveyed adequately by language.

However, there is a record of the self-realization or liberation of a seventeen-year-old Indian schoolboy who was living in his parents' house in 1896. He had undergone no spiritual training nor had he learned anything of yoga or spiritual philosophy before this event. This is how he described it later:

It was about six weeks before I left Madura for good that the great change in my life took place. It was quite sudden. I was sitting alone in a room on the first floor of my uncle's house. I seldom had any sickness, and on that day there was nothing wrong with my health, but a sudden violent fear of death overtook me.

There was nothing in my state of health to account for it, and I did not try to account for it or to find out whether there was any reason for the fear. I just felt 'I am going to die' and began thinking what to do about it. It did not occur to me to consult a doctor or my elders or friends; I felt I had to solve the problem myself, there and then.

The shock of the fear of death drove my mind inwards and I said to myself mentally, without actually framing the words: 'Now death has come; what does it mean? What is it that is dying? This body dies.' And I at once dramatized the occurrence of death. I lay with my limbs stretched out stiff, as though rigor mortis had set in, and imitated a corpse so as to give greater reality to the enquiry. I held my breath and kept my lips tightly closed so that no sound could escape, so that neither the word 'I' nor any other word could be uttered. 'Well then,' I said to myself, 'this body is dead. It will be carried stiff to the burning ground and there burnt and reduced to ashes. But with the death of this body am I dead? Is the body 'I'? It is silent and inert but I feel the full force of my personality and even the voice of the 'I' within me, apart from it. So I am Spirit transcending the body. The body dies but the Spirit transcending it cannot be touched by death. This means I am the deathless Spirit.'

All this was not dull thought; it flashed through me vividly, almost without thought process. 'I' was something very real, the only real thing about my present state, and all the conscious activity connected with my body was centred on that 'I'. From that moment onwards the 'I', or Self, focused attention on itself by a powerful fascination. Fear of death had vanished once and for all.

A few weeks after this event the young man, who was later given the name Ramana Maharshi, made a pilgrimage to the holy hill of Arunachala and stayed there for the next fifty-four years, meditating and teaching mainly through silence.

Ramana Maharshi's near-death experience forced him to come face to face with death, and this confrontation brought on a spiritual awakening about the nature of life. He realized that in death it was only his body that would die; his real Self would be unaffected by his death.

As the *Aitreya Upanishad* says,

Who is the Self that we meditate on? Is it the Self by which we see, hear, smell, taste and through which we speak? Is Self the mind by which we perceive, understand, know, remember, will, desire and love? These are but servants of the true Self who is pure consciousness. This Self is everything in everything. People who realize this Eternal Self live in joy and go beyond death.

This insight is the kind of knowledge that yoga seeks, a subjective knowledge which cannot be tested in a laboratory but is 'proved' internally, in the sense that the liberated person intuitively knows and feels the truth. This is essential or fundamental truth, the truth that relates to the essence of who we are. As the *Katha Upanishad* says,

The light of the Eternal Spirit is invisible and hidden in everyone. It is seen only by those who keep their mind concentrated on love and thus develop a super conscious manner of knowing. Meditation enables them to go deeper and deeper into consciousness, from the world of words to the world of thoughts and then beyond thoughts to the wisdom in the Self, finding inner peace.

In our post-modern age we hold truth to be relative, but the truth of yoga is considered to be an absolute knowledge of the inner and timeless Self. And the yogis say that with this knowledge come a fearlessness and security which hold even death at bay.

Not many of us will undergo a one-off life-changing experience like Ramana Maharshi's, and perhaps we wouldn't want to. But life is constantly changing, and we can only help ourselves by choosing a spiritual path that encourages and enables positive change. The ultimate aim of yoga is a transformed mind, one that sees the world clearly, as it really is, not distorted by the illusions that normally cloud our vision. It is not that yoga imposes a new way of looking at the world from the outside. Rather, it wipes away the errors that screen us from seeing it correctly, in the same way that we wipe accumulated dirt from a window to let the light shine in.

This is a similar process to Michelangelo's fanciful theory of sculpting. We usually think that a sculptor carves away at a rough block of marble to make it resemble a shape that he holds in his imagination. But Michelangelo half-jokingly said that the shape was already in the marble, waiting to be let out. His job was just to carve away the excess and let the marble reveal the shape. Michelangelo's art was not in creating the figure but in liberating it. This is also the way of yoga, a means of liberating our Self by removing all the rubbish that has accumulated around it. It is a negative process leading to a positive result, a way of making progress by going into reverse.

The new vision of the world that yoga reveals brings with it an opening of the heart, so that we begin to feel a tenderness that extends itself from us to envelop all of creation. We feel a deep connection with everything that lives, and our understanding of what lives includes things that we formerly thought were dead matter, like stones and stars.

This expansion of our emotions is a religious feeling, which does not need a belief in God to be expressed. Although yoga has traditionally been theistic, it comes from a Hindu tradition that does not discriminate between believers and atheists. Since yoga pre-dates Hinduism, it is not tied to any one religion, so is applicable to any religious faith, or none at all. A belief in God is not necessary for the practice of yoga, but I have found that one of the results of yoga is a profound feeling that I can only call religious. Yoga induces in me (and others) a feeling of the sacred, by giving us the experience of a unity, a oneness, with everything else. Since this feeling of oneness is difficult to achieve, those who manage to find it hold yoga in the highest esteem.

3

Yoga as a Tool

If you've ever had the pleasure of owning a new pair of walking boots, you know the lovely delicate sensation of unwrapping them from their soft tissue paper covering and holding them admiringly in your hands, the soft and supple leather smooth to the touch. You slip the strong and solid boots on your thickly stockinged feet and anticipate the satisfaction of sloshing through cold deep puddles and slimy mud, secure in the knowledge that your boots will not let you down, and that your feet, sheathed and sealed, can trample through the worst conditions without becoming cold and wet.

But when you return home from your walk, those beautiful new boots are caked with dried mud and leaves, and the deeply corrugated soles and heels are heavily encrusted with a mixture of pebbles, twigs and hard baked earth which can't be easily dislodged. To prise out this toughened debris we need to use a tool, a strong and sensitive blade of some kind, to lever out the coagulated mess and enable the boots to return, not to that perfection that we first uncovered in the soft tissue, but at least to a clean and dry state fit for the next outing.

We are like those boots, pristine and perfect when we first emerge from the womb, but the dust of life on earth clings to us as soon as we are handled by our parents, and as we move through life, as we mature and grow, our conditioning and experiences allow more dust and dirt to stick to us, leaving us heavier than we were, less shiny and pure. The yogis call these impurities of life kleshas, toxins clogging up our system, both physical and spiritual. Like the boots, which need a cleaning tool to return them to a state fit for use, we too are in need of a tool to return us to a state of fitness. To me, yoga is such a tool.

By the time most of us come to yoga our bodies have been damaged, sometimes quite badly, by life and civilization. Modern life, with its car culture, sedentary yet frenetic life-style, stressful work-places, polluted air, water and processed food contributes to produce bodies that are stiff, inflexible, often overweight, and generally unhealthy. Our bodies also harbour the lasting effect of negative emotions like pain, sorrow, grief, fear, loss and anger. Physically, mentally and spiritually strained, our bodies are just waiting to incubate the diseases of the West – cancer and heart disease.

Many people breathe shallowly and only from the chest, not realizing that the whole body is itself a respiratory organ and that failure to breathe properly inhibits the body from its proper physiological function. We often have our toes cramped and feet narrowed from years of being squeezed into fashionable shoes, and our spines either bent or stuck due to a combination of poor postural habits and badly designed seating. Most of us walk incorrectly, holding our heads either too far forward or too far back, often hunching our shoulders and neck. Many of us have joints that are stiff and lack movement and flexibility.

This poor state of our bodies is usually mirrored by the state of our minds, and our souls – if we can locate them – are often plagued by fear and insecurity, alienating us from others. We find it hard to show compassion towards strangers, are often less than loving to those we live with, can be selfish with money, and thoughtlessly hurt others through emotional shut-down or by acting rashly and angrily out of our own fear and insecurity. Worse still, we often fail in loving ourselves and feel less than confident about our own intrinsic worth.

This distorted state of body, mind and spirit is characterized by the Sanskrit term *duhkha*, which is usually translated as suffering or anguish. The first Noble Truth of that greatest of yogis, the Buddha, was that all life is duhkha – suffering or pain. The idea that life is unsatisfactory, full of pain, suffering and anguish, is a basic Indian view, shared by all the Indian philosophies. This anguish comes not only from the ordinary difficulties of life that we all share, but also from the Indians' unique view of the world.

The ancient Indian sages believed that the universe was eternal, with no beginning and end, an everlasting cycle – the wheel of life. In this constant round of existence, each being was destined to be reborn repeatedly, forced to live out their individual cycle of birth and death forever. If we consider one lifetime to be full of difficulties, how would we feel about having to repeat unsatisfactory lives endlessly, with no possibility of escape? The sages believed this cycle of eternal pain and frustration could only be broken by gaining moksha or liberation, the state in which one realizes that one's true Self is deathless and eternal, and with this knowledge one escapes from having to be reborn again. The cycle of samsara, of birth and rebirth, is thereby broken.

In the West we have never believed in an eternally revolving, beginning-less universe. The Judeo-Christian tradition is that God created the universe at a specific time, and at some time in the future it will come to an end. Our science backs this up with the theory of the Big Bang, a violent explosion that started the universe, time and space at a specific moment in the past. Our theology, philosophy and science lead us to see time as linear and not cyclical, and to believe that the world has an historic dimension, a place where there is a past, a present and a future. Each individual Western life is finite, limited in time and place, and death represents an ending, a rounding off of experience.

To those who believe in Jesus, his martyrdom provides salvation for their souls, which will live on after death in heaven (or hell). But for those who do not believe in Christianity, or can no longer convince themselves that their souls live on, death is the ultimate conclusion and the final separation. I believe that fear of death is the bottom-line fear in contemporary culture, and all the other fears we have – of poverty, illness or loneliness – are off-shoots of this primary and fundamental terror.

Some people seem to be able to cope with this finality of life's extinction. They believe that life is dominated entirely by chance, and human life is merely an accident of nature without any possibility of meaning. They are willing to live with the strongest possible doubt that there is any higher power, order or purpose to life. They have abandoned traditional religion as irrelevant and feel no need to seek alternative forms of spirituality. This kind of tough-minded existential position, so very post-modern, does not feel the need for any emotional 'crutch' of religion or salvation to lean on, or a spiritual band-aid to make life more bearable by believing in something extra-rational to provide spiritual comfort when we need it.

When things are going well, and health, money and relationships are satisfactory, this kind of materialistic attitude is fine, but if work or love affairs turn sour, or unexpected death or illness strikes, there seems to be very little positive reinforcement available from this viewpoint, to shore up accelerating unhappiness. This tough-minded view of a life without meaning might then turn quite bleak and dark, since most people are incapable of living for long with a high level of doubt, especially if it turns into despair.

In Roman times, the Stoic philosophers said that when

life becomes too painful or difficult, there is always an exit route – suicide. If you found life intolerable, you could always end it, as Seneca wrote:

> *Epicurus said, 'Think of death.' The meaning is clear – that it is a wonderful thing to learn thoroughly how to die. In saying this, he bids us think of freedom. The person who has learned to die has unlearned slavery; he is beyond any external power. What terrors have prisons and chains and bars for him? His way out is clear. There is only one chain which binds us to life, and that is the love of life. This chain may not be cast off, but it may be rubbed away, so that, when necessity shall demand, nothing may retard or hinder us from being ready to do at once that which at some time we are bound to do.*

We don't share this attitude, but believe that unhappiness and misery can be turned around and life transformed through various kinds of therapy – mental, physical and spiritual. It's remarkable that our positive attitude to change, an aspect of the Western belief in material progress, coincides with an Eastern view of spiritual progress – that the mind is the source of suffering and that it is capable of complete alteration. After all, the Buddha's Third Noble Truth is that suffering can be brought to an end.

What strikes me most strongly about the Indian attitude to philosophy and spirituality is its insistence on seeking the truth, and belief that the truth can be found, no matter how difficult that search may be or where it may lead. Here is one of the major differences between East and West. The Western mind searches the external world for information to discover practical answers to the fundamental questions of existence, but the Indian mind has always searched inwards, not for practical information for its own sake but for transformation. The discovery of the Self, that timeless and changeless

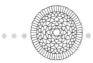

essence at the heart of our individual life, is the Indians'
prized discovery.

Perhaps the marriage of the West's material progress and
the East's spiritual progress may be the unity that we are
looking for in the twenty-first century.

4

Patanjali's Classical Yoga System

The *Yoga Sutras*, scholars tell us, were written sometime during the period from the fourth to the third century BCE. No more accurate dating is available since ancient Indian history lacks secure dates on which to pin the major literary and philosophical texts. The word *sutra* means thread, as in linking thoughts, the way we say, 'I lost the thread.' A sutra contains a number of linking thoughts about a subject expressed quite tersely, without elucidation, and so normally needs a commentary to explain it. That commentary then invites a further commentary and so it goes on *ad infinitum*.

Little is known of Patanjali, who compiled the *Sutras*, other than to assume that he was stitching together diverse material about yoga that had been in existence in oral form for many hundreds of years before he gathered it into a single text. The *Yoga Sutras* form the basis of yoga philosophy, one of the six schools of Indian philosophy, and its core beliefs informed Buddhist philosophy.

Patanjali's text concentrates on Raja Yoga, which means royal or kingly yoga. This is a form of yoga concerned with controlling the mind mainly through meditation, unlike the much later Hatha Yoga, the form of yoga mostly practised in the West, which developed more fully asanas and pranayama, the physical positions and breath control. The *Yoga Sutras* do not describe specific asanas or pranayama but concentrate instead on the psychological and spiritual aspects of yoga. The focus is on silencing thoughts, so that an inner peace prevails, in which the Self, our true nature, can be discovered and realized.

In the early days of yoga, the asanas were less important for physical exercise and were intended for purposes of meditation. The classic asana for meditation is the Lotus position, with the legs crossed, one foot placed on top of the opposite thigh, the hands placed on the knees facing upwards, and the thumb and first finger touching. In this position the body becomes so comfortably seated and firmly locked on the floor that it allows the mind and emotions to quieten, and pranayama exercises and then meditation can be performed. This is how it is described in the *Shvetashvatara Upanishad*:

> *The wise person holds his body straight, with head, neck and chest in line, withdraws his mind and senses towards the heart, and on the raft of the spirit crosses safely through dangerous waters.*
>
> *Subduing all activity and regulating his breath, the wise person breathes in and out gently through the nostrils. Let him control his mind, which is like a chariot pulled by wild horses.*

Patanjali says that yoga practice is the means to still the mind, thereby allowing the inner Self, our true ruler, to become isolated in itself and to find liberation:

> *Yoga is when the Self rests in its own being, in our own original nature which is pure awareness.*

Yoga is a means by which we can gain subtle and discriminating knowledge, a wisdom that is hard to come by when following our ordinary way of living. One of the most difficult of all the distinctions we have to make is to clarify the confusion between what is the real Self and what is the mind. This confusion lies at the heart of much of our perplexity:

The human Self is under the power of the forces of nature, and thus it falls into confusion. Because of this confusion the Self cannot become conscious of the Spirit who dwells within and whose power gives us the power to act. The Self is thus whirled along the rushing stream of muddy waters of the forces of nature and becomes unsteady and wavering, filled with confusion and full of desires, lacking concentration and disturbed with pride.

If we can separate our little self, our ego, from our true Self within, which is Spirit, we can attain discriminating knowledge, and the wisdom of the heart will spontaneously flower. We then understand intuitively and naturally just who we truly are and what it is that we truly need. This inner truth is Self-realization, the height of yoga training.

One of the goals of yoga is a steady and tranquil mind, since a continuing sense of calm and tranquillity allows healthy energies to accumulate. Yoga aims at altering our heady life of thinking, our rational mind, which is based on the brain's frontal lobes and normally seeks external knowledge, into a mind that can experience a different kind of internal knowledge. Since unsteadiness of mind is the main hurdle to acquiring this experience, yoga aims to steady the mind so it can be concentrated exclusively on the Self and not on the outside objects that it normally attaches to. By withdrawing the senses inwards we try to break this attachment.

Patanjali's theory about the isolation of the Self differs from a teaching often quoted in yoga books which says that the union yoga seeks is a merging of our individual

Self with the Supreme Self, Brahman or God. This is the philosophy of another of the Indian schools, the Vedanta, and the reason why it is so often quoted is that most of the Indian yogis who taught in the West were followers of Advaita Vedanta philosophy, the most influential of all the Indian philosophies, and the one adhered to by most educated Hindus. The Swamis Vivekananda, Shivananda, Muktananda, Satchidananda, Parahamsa Yogananda, and Vishnu-devananda all are or were Advaita Vedantists and consequently taught this philosophy to their students and promulgated it in their writings.

Patanjali's yoga philosophy differs from that of the Advaita Vedantists not only in yoga's idea of the isolation of the Self. To Patanjali the Self and the world are both real and have a real existence, whereas for the Vedantists the world is unreal, being a manifestation of maya, or illusion. I don't want to get too bogged down in a philosophical squabble, but I think it's worth trying to clarify this point, otherwise a confusion that is very widespread will continue.

People are often under the impression that Hindu philosophy believes that the world is an illusion, a dream, an appearance or an hallucination. It is just a play, or lila, of God, created by Brahman, the Supreme Self or Divine principle. The phenomenal world is seen as a kind of movie, which is unreal, but when we are ignorant and do not realize this, we believe it to be real.

A real-life movie example can illuminate this. One of the first film screenings ever held was in Paris at the turn of the twentieth century. People had never seen a moving picture, so when there was a scene of a speeding train pulling into a station, spectators panicked and ran out of their seats, fearing for their lives. They took the illusion for reality and reacted wrongly out of ignorance. The Vedantists say that our worldly life, like the movie, is an illusion, and that Brahman, the Supreme Self, is like a film director who creates this appearance and presents it to us. In our ignorance we think this movie of life is real and so we take it seriously, suffering under its terms and conditions. But if we become liberated, through yoga, we realize that it is only an illusion and has no reality or meaning whatsoever. It is just an entertainment.

The Vedantists say that the only true reality is Brahman, the eternal and unchanging principle. Everything else is a manifestation of Brahman, and is consequently not real, but an illusion. Since the world, and everything in it, is not real, the aim of yoga, for the Advaita, is to wake up from this dream and become liberated from it. This allows us to realize our true Self, called Atman. We discover that Atman, the inner Self, is as real as Brahman because the two are alike, and the aim of yoga is for the Atman and the Brahman to merge. The Vedantists also call this merging Self-realization, and it represents the complete identification of the Self with God, Brahman. This teaching of the Advaita Vedantists has its basis in the *Upanishads*, the ancient speculative philo-sophical texts of India. The following passage is from the *Chandogya Upanishad*:

> *The whole universe comes from the highest Spirit, Brahman, and will return to the Spirit. In silence we must direct our deepest desires with prayers, faith and vision to the Spirit, Brahman, to realize our Self.*
>
> *The Self that dwells in our hearts is the Self that can only be realized in the silence of understanding that we are but Spirit, and that our minds and hearts must be truthful and pure, finding, beyond words, joy in the essence of our being.*
>
> *This Self who gives rise to all works, desire, odours, tastes and who embraces the whole universe, who is beyond words, who is pure joy and who is always in your heart is the higher Spirit, Brahman. When my ego dies and finds its restful place, I will find him.*

The Vedantists consider the coming together of Atman and Brahman, the individual Self merging with the Supreme Self, as the ultimate aim of yoga. Since the Atman and Brahman are effectively the same, it implies that the individual Self is pure Spirit and is therefore identical with Brahman, God. The *Chandogya Upanishad* teaches this identity:

> *There is nothing in the cosmos that doesn't come from that one Being. Of everything that exists, this Being is the inner-most Self. He is the truth, the Self Supreme. And you are that!*
>
> *Even though we cannot see it, the Self is within all things and there is nothing that doesn't come from Him.*
>
> *This invisible and subtle essence is the Spirit of the whole universe. That is reality. That is truth. And you are that!*

The well-known saying of the Vedantists 'You are that' means that you and the universe are the same, that your consciousness and that of the universe are the same consciousness, and since the universe is God, you too are God-like. The Vedanta philosophy is a monistic and absolutist one, believing that there exists only one reality, the one without a second, that of the Divine Brahman merged with the Atman. Brahman is unseen and can't be felt or heard, but it is the power and primary principle that spontaneously manifests itself as the foundation of all creation. It is also spiritual in nature, so the Vedantists consider the entire universe as Spirit, as the *Upanishads* state:

> *The Eternal Spirit is everywhere, to the left of you, to the right of you, above and below, in front and behind. What is this world but Spirit?*
>
> *Everything is based on Spirit; Spirit is the foundation of the universe, Spirit is Brahman.*

But Patanjali's yoga philosophy doesn't believe this. It believes that the world of nature is a real world, not a mask of illusion. Patanjali does not believe that the world is an hallucination, so he has no interest in freeing us from the illusion that the world is a dream. He sees yoga's goal as freeing us from a different illusion – that we are the same as our body, mind and senses. As A. G. Mohan says,

> *for most people the body is the primary object of which we are aware, so that most of us identify 'Self' in some way with our physical being. We experience ourselves, our environment and other people through our bodies.*

Because of the nature of perception, we mistakenly identify ourselves with the phenomenal world, and fail to understand that our real identity is not with our body or mind but with our true Self. To isolate and realize that Self is the aim of classical yoga. And for Patanjali our experience of the world only makes sense if we admit the equal and independent reality of Nature and Spirit.

Patanjali's philosophy is not monist, believing in only one being or reality, but dualistic. He believes that there exists not one singular reality, Brahman, but two realities which are opposed – Nature and Spirit – that none the less work together in a kind of marriage. Nature is material, it forms our body, mind and senses and is forever churning and changing over time, while the Spirit is our inner Self – formless, changeless and eternal. Working together through daily experience, nature and spirit enable us over time to discover the true nature of reality.

I think Patanjali presents his philosophy in this dual way because it mirrors how we ordinarily perceive the world. Our usual way of looking at the world is to assume a separation and difference between our subjective being and the objective world. Patanjali explains in the *Sutras* that this normal perception is really false and displays avidya, which he calls ignorance, and this seems to be our starting position. Perhaps he thought it best to describe the world as we see it, so that we are able to understand our erroneous view and discover, through yoga, how to replace our confusion and ignorance with true knowledge.

5

How We See the World

The problem of our false perception of Self is due to our normal common-sense way of looking at things. We believe that the world is made up of separate individual objects and that each object exists in itself, although it has relationships with other objects. The structure of our language is based on this view of the world as well, since we say, for example, 'I see the apple.' I, a subjective individual, see something, an object, an oval red fruit. In our world subjects do things to objects and vice versa. We believe that the world is real and that it is made up of real interacting objects.

Well, isn't the world made up of real objects? Not according to Jeremy Hayward in his book *Letters to Vanessa*. He explains that common sense gives us the impression that our eyes are like cameras that merely reproduce what exists 'out there' in the world. Unfortunately, common sense is quite wrong about what is going on 'out there'.

When someone blind from birth manages to have their sight restored, they do not immediately see the world we see. What happens first is that they are overwhelmed with light, which their sensitive eyes cannot endure without being heavily shaded. Our minds have adapted to this glare to enable us to cope with the intense brightness, which we can no longer see. But the newly sighted person, even after learning to adapt to this intense light, still sees no objects. There is only a chaos of impressions and light, and for this person to see an apple as an object takes a great deal of visual education, learning to see our world.

Our eyes do not reproduce what is 'out there'. Instead, it is our mind that creates what is out there, based on what we have been taught to expect to find. When we look at something, our retina may reflect a solid object, but what the optic nerve sends to the brain is a set of signals or impulses, which our mind needs to decode, identify and interpret. The act of interpretation is mixed up with all the values that have been implanted in us by society, and we are unable to 'see' anything without that image being accompanied by both a feeling and a judgment about it. We don't see anything objectively; only through a subjective film, a film of desire informing our vision. Seeing is a creative act, not an imitative one. We are not cameras but artists, and the world is our canvas.

According to the physicists, what is 'out there' is just waves of light, an integrated and intelligent pattern of energy, constantly moving and altering. Everything in the universe is composed of electrons, protons and neutrons, dancing in endlessly altering patterns. Following Einstein, who explained that the forms of solid matter that we see are just whirls of energy, scientists have learned that the universe is composed of energy fields, without any 'real' solidity.

If we can imagine the world without form, without forms of colour or forms of sound, but merely as sets of vibrations and waves, we can begin to understand the saying of the Chinese Chan Buddhists,

Form is emptiness
Emptiness is form.

The forms of things that we see and hear are really empty of form. It is our nervous system and our brains that create this world of form. Without the form that our minds impose on the world, the world is only a collection of waves or vibrations, patterns that relate to each other. And since we are also in this world, we too are just so many relating waves and oscillations. What we encounter is not the world itself, since all we can experience of it is our own nervous system.

Our minds create the solidity of objects, add colour to them and organize them in three-dimensional space, thereby creating a visual field that makes sense to us. In this field we place ourselves, satisfied that we now 'exist' in real time and in real space. We make a distinction between living and non-living things that goes against the physicist's view of the world, for all things are alive with atoms, and it makes little sense to discriminate between things in this way. But our life is dominated by discrimination of all kinds, preferences for one thing over another, for one way of acting over another. It is through these discriminations and preferences that we become attached to objects, ideas and feelings.

Under the illusion that the world is composed of 'real' objects, we create a 'real' self to interact with them. The *Yoga Sutras* explain that our common-sense way of perceiving the world creates in us an ego-centred mind, the 'I/me', which we feel we need to establish, to confront a 'real' world. First we create a false identity and then we identify with it as our self. This is the mask, the false image of ourselves that seeks pleasure and avoids pain, the ego-driven self that wants to deny the possibility of illness and death. This limited self pursues endless selfish desires, and wants to use the objects of the world to satisfy these desires. It is the basis of our personality, our persona.

Patanjali says that because our ego-driven mind is mainly interested in pursuing selfish desires, it views and interprets the world according to these desires, and so falls into a confused state, a state of delusion in which it misconceives what the world is really like. He calls this state avidya – ignorance. This is a condition in which we lack wisdom because we have the illusion that our vision of the world is a correct one, even though we suffer because of it. We really experience spiritual darkness, bound by our desires. Yoga philosophy believes that the mind itself is not spiritual but part of nature, of matter, and that is why our thoughts have a real force in the world. If we hold erroneous thoughts, we act in erroneous ways, and this causes us to suffer, because we are not seeing the world clearly. We have a false vision of life, and it is this false view of things that causes our difficulties.

The way to change that false view to a correct one, to lose avidya and gain true knowledge, is by allowing the source of our knowledge – the inner Self – to radiate the light of its knowledge through our mind and body. The true Self, according to Patanjali, sits eternally as a calm, patient, silent and radiant witness beyond the mind. According to the *Sutras*, the Spirit does nothing, it is just a silent observer that sees everything that takes place. It is light, a light that shines through the mind, body and beyond. This light is the true Self that we seek, but, paradoxically, there is no need to seek it, because the sages say it is always there, waiting silently. We only need to discover it, and to uncover it, so that its light can radiate with no obstructions.

Patanjali talks of avidya as a kind of veil that blocks this light from reaching the mind, and I think of it as a kind of fog of confusion that gathers between the mind and the Self, obstructing the Self's radiance. Consequently the object of yoga is to pierce this veil, dissolve the fog, so that the Self and the mind are once again in direct and clear communication. Once this happens, the false, deluded vision is replaced by a truer vision.

I am a concrete thinker, and not a very good abstract one; I need to consider things as visible and actual before I feel that I truly understand them. So for my own understanding I need to construct a home for the Self, a home in my body where I can imagine it resting.

In Tai Chi we locate the chi energy – the life energy –
somewhere below the navel in a place called the Tan Tien,
and in yoga this same life energy is the prana which travels
in channels all around the spine and eventually up and down
it when the kundalini energy is released. My own preference
for a place in the body that houses the Self is the solar plexus,
which I identify with the heart, and with the earliest form
of brain, the reptilian brain. I think this is the first place in
our body where we are aware of feelings – 'aware' being too
subtle a word for what is a basic and direct visceral reaction,
a wrenching of the guts. We feel the strongest emotions here,
and we also feel that this is the home of our intuition. So
the solar plexus is where I locate my Self or Spirit. The
Chandogya Upanishad also locates the Spirit in the heart:

> *In the centre of the castle of the infinite Spirit, which is
> Brahman, in our own body, there is a small shrine shaped like
> a lotus flower in which there is a small space. We need to find
> out who lives there and we should desire to know Him. Why
> is it so important?*
>
> *Because this little space within our hearts is as great as
> the whole vast world outside. Heaven, earth, fire, wind, the
> sun, moon and stars; whatever is and whatever is not, every-
> thing is there, for the whole universe is in Him and He dwells
> in our hearts.*
>
> *The Spirit that lives in that space does not grow old and
> die. No one can ever kill the Spirit that is everlasting. The love
> of the universe dwells in the real castle of the Spirit, which
> we call Brahman.*

Having found a home in the middle of my body for the
Self/Spirit, I locate my ego, the 'I/me', in my head, especially
the frontal lobes, where I do all the rational and conscious
thinking that leads me away from my heart and my feelings.
If the 'I/me' is dominated by this kind of abstract and linear

thinking and loses its connection to the heart, it eventually becomes arid and death-like.

When we operate from the selfish and limited ego, there is a separation between the head and the heart, and this division leads to the feeling that we are pulled in two directions at once. Our heart may want to offer compassion to people, but our head fears being taken advantage of. Our heart may want to help those who are suffering, but our head says be realistic – this is the way life is. We are constantly torn between two ways of acting, and this split – the divided Self – leads us into a disharmony of spirit.

Yoga represents a method of creating harmony out of disharmony and of reintegrating our head with our heart, our body with our mind, to establish spiritual health. The end result of yoga is not just to feel this union of head and heart, body and spirit, but also to experience the joy of that union. It is this joy that we want to find, since joy or bliss in living is really the supreme spiritual enlightenment.

6

The Ashtanga System

Patanjali's *Yoga Sutras* are a kind of self-help manual to help us dissolve our ignorance, gain true wisdom and find joy in living. The *Sutras* explain the theory behind the method of all types of yoga, which Patanjali describes as an ashtanga system. Ashtanga means eight-limbed, and each limb constitutes one part of the practice, although all the parts must be practised simultaneously for it to be really yoga. By a limb Patanjali means the limb of a tree or of a person, a living, growing organism.

Yoga is not a theoretical system but a practical one, in which the practice must lead to an end result: a new way of looking at the world. I like to think of it as a form of cooking, in which many ingredients are used for an end result that can only be satisfyingly tested by taste. Patanjali's ashtanga system can be considered as eight ingredients of a recipe for a magnificent cake, and I would like to discuss it in those terms.

Now, I've never baked a cake myself, but I have helped to decorate a few. If I had to make one on my own, I would probably consult a cookbook and carefully follow one of its recipes. By doing this, I might successfully bake an edible cake. But if I decided to ignore this resource and just proceed with my own ideas, it's likely that I would miss out a key ingredient, like eggs, and produce a hard, dry, crumbly, inedible mess.

This kind of half-baked cooking may be where contemporary yoga is heading, since Patanjali's eight-part yoga recipe seems to be ignored by many teachers and practitioners of yoga. The yoga taught today in many fitness centres and gyms leaves out a number of key ingredients which have been tested for hundreds of years, and which have provided an effective plan for personal development. Instead of being grateful to Patanjali for having given us such a detailed recipe, we are casually dropping from practice some of his key points. In doing so, we are losing sight of the ultimate goal and becoming obsessed with only a few of the techniques leading to it. If we continue in this way, the West may lose the essence of yoga and replace it with just another fitness regime for the body.

The ingredients for a delicious and satisfying yoga 'cake', according to Patanjali, are these eight, which can be broken into three groups:

1. Yama 2. Niyama	Ethical and Spiritual Practices
3. Asana 4. Pranayama	Physical Practices
5. Pratyahara 6. Dharana 7. Dhayana 8. Samadhi	Meditation Practices

7

Ethical and Spiritual Training

Yama and niyama represent the spiritual side of our nature in relation to the three dimensions of the Self. The first dimension is how we see ourselves – I and I; the second is how we see others – I and you; and the third is how we relate to the universe at large – I and You or I and It. Yoga practice enables us to become more aware of our attitude to these three relationships and helps us to re-integrate our vision of life, so that these three dimensions of the Self enter into a unity, a oneness.

Unfortunately, the ethical and spiritual teachings of Patanjali are the ones that are most often dropped out of the Western yoga mix. This is partly because they touch on personal morality, something which many people feel is an entirely private matter and not something to be discussed in a yoga class. Similarly, yoga instructors may not feel confident about raising subjects of an ethical nature and are more secure teaching positions and breathing, the more obvious physical side.

But Patanjali says that the ethical and spiritual teachings are of equal importance to the others and need to be lived if a true transformation and liberation are to take place. I would like to explain what yama and niyama mean to me, why they are essential, and how they can be used in yoga practice.

There are five aspects each to yama and niyama,

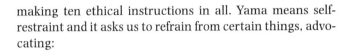

making ten ethical instructions in all. Yama means self-restraint and it asks us to refrain from certain things, advocating:

1. non-violence
2. non-lying
3. not-stealing
4. sexual moderation
5. not being greedy

Niyama means personal observance and its aspects are more positive in that it wants us to act in certain way, aiming for:

1. purity
2. contentment
3. discipline
4. study
5. devotion

Of these ten ethical teachings, half are things we must not do, and half are things we should do. We have come across ten precepts like this in our own culture, when Moses came down from Mount Sinai bearing the Ten Commandments of YHWH (God). These commandments have a certain similarity to Patanjali's:

1. You must have no other God besides me.
2. You must not make or pray to idols.
3. You must not use the name of God for evil intent.
4. Hold the Sabbath day holy.
5. Honour your father and your mother.
6. You must not commit murder.
7. You must not commit adultery.
8. You must not steal.

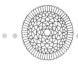

9. You must not lie.
10. You must not covet.

Of the Ten Hebrew Commandments, eight are expressed as a negative 'You must not' and only two are positive. Of the negative ones, the last five commandments – not to murder, commit adultery, steal, lie and covet – are almost exactly equivalent to the five yama self-restraints. What this surely tells us is that if two distinct philosophies separated so absolutely by culture, location, time and language have devised exactly the same teachings, there must be something to them.

Yoga philosophy believes that our inner Self is identical to all other selves, and when we look into another person's (or animal's) eyes we are looking directly at their Self, which is also our Self, as the *Isha Upanishad* states:

> *When we can see the Spirit in others, we feel no fear because we understand that we are all one. When we have this sense of unity, there is nothing that we can delude ourselves with, and we feel no sorrow or grief. We are all filled with the same light and innocence.*

So when we act in the world, our actions seem to be directed at others, but in truth they are directed at our own Self. Not only that, but the unity of life means that all these ethical teachings intermingle, so that they are not separate items of behaviour but are interdependent. If our behaviour is positive, our actions reinforce each other in a healthy and wholesome manner, a cycle of goodness and benevolence, but if we act negatively, they feed into each other with increasingly corrosive moral effects, a downward cycle of ultimate despair.

The yamas show us all the erroneous behaviour that we exhibit when we are in the grip of avidya – ignorance. These negative acts are symptoms of spiritual darkness, of a lack of wisdom. They result from our belief that we can acquire happiness through desiring external things, especially when that desire is expressed as a wish that our life could be better. When we think that by acquiring things we will acquire happiness, we invariably enter into a downward cycle of desire, leading to frustration, leading to anger, culminating in pain for ourself and others.

The yamas all exhibit the negative side of selfish desire: greed to have more than others, stealing as a way to achieve this, lying and violence to get our way, and sexual exploitation for personal needs.

Patanjali wants us to change the way we act, because changing our actions is the outer spiritual work of yoga, which accompanies the inner spiritual work of meditation. The aim is not to have a mind obsessed with desires, pulled every which way by the attractions of pleasure and the aversions of pain, but a steady and harmonious mind, one that can look on the world with a measure of tranquillity, and see clearly what our place is, and how we should act. So the yamas also show a positive side, the attitude and behaviour that a yogi takes to these same impulses.

The Yamas / Self-restraint

Non-violence means not harming, injuring or hurting another creature, and therefore means offering compassion and love both to ourselves and to others. The yogi knows that all creatures are his one Self, that in his essence he is no different from others and so must treat them with exactly the same respect as he does himself. This is really just another instance of the Golden Rule.

But when we act from the deluded ego-driven self, life is totally different. We normally live out a negative cycle: from fear comes insecurity, from insecurity comes craving or greed, from greed comes frustration, from frustration comes anger, and from anger comes aggression and violence – leading to separation and ugliness.

The yogi, by freeing himself from fear and insecurity, has no need to attach himself to outside objects and does not go down this negative spiral, but creates a positive one, leading to unity and beauty. By not acting in a negative, aggressive, violent way, he creates an atmosphere in which everyone he comes into contact with feels this harmonious and peaceful atmosphere and responds positively to it. He creates around himself a state of peace and harmony in which he can respond freely and creatively in everything he does.

This precept gives us a clue as to how to get the best out of those we come into contact with. If we are not aggressive, almost all the people we meet will be equally non-threatening, and those who approach us with aggression will feel quite disarmed by our lack of aggressive response. What we give out to the world returns to us, and we all know that when we are angry or aggressive, we meet rage around every corner.

Non-violence seems to be the only attitude with the chance to heal our hurting, damaged world. If we continue to fight each other with weapons of mass destruction, and have no conscience about how we exploit and destroy the environment, we will continue the cycle of darkness and destruction that has haunted our so-called civilization and could destroy it completely. Non-violence to ourselves, to others and to the earth is the only philosophy that has a chance to regenerate our culture. Non-violence is a radical belief, one that overturns tens of thousands of years of blind anger, revenge and hatred. No doubt this is why people find it so difficult to put into practice.

Not lying, truthfulness, means to be true to your inner Self and to express your heart's truth openly and freely in speech and action. When thoughts, words and deeds are all one, we live an integrated life and are part of the unity that we feel all around us. The truth has a power that we are able to use consciously and unconsciously to further everything we do.

But this is not how the deluded mind works. Ignorance means that our Self is divided, and the contradictions of this confused ego bring out lies, deceptions and denial as tools to paper over cracks in the Self. Life becomes more complicated and stressful as we try to remember what lies we have told, and to whom. Since we already have far too much stress to deal with, why add more? This straightforward approach to life avoids harming those we lie to, and being simply truthful brings with it a great self-respect and confidence. Telling the truth has a further benefit in that you become more - sensitive to the truth and can detect when someone is lying to you.

Mahatma Gandhi thought so highly of these first two yamas – non-violence and truth – that he modelled his life and political programme on them. Although it is easy to think of them as too idealistic to put into practice, Gandhi's example, and his achievement in gaining Indian Independence in 1948, prove that these are realistic as well as idealistic methods. Gandhi believed that the truth was God, and that if a person lived his or her own truth with absolute integrity and honesty, this truth would bring them into the closest possible connection with the God they respected and worshipped.

Non-stealing means what it says. We all know not to take goods, money or property belonging to others, but do we also consider what it means inconsiderately to take more subtle things like attention, affection, time or goodwill? Sexual relations are fraught with people stealing affection and love from others, with no intention of returning it. In business, people may not steal outright, but they use their positions of power or knowledge to carve out deals that are so advantageous that they amount to legal theft. Our global economy, that is structurally so weighted to the benefit of the Western world, is seen by the poor Third World as organized theft.

Stealing of any kind is obviously a potent form of harm and violence, and if at the same time we deny the reality of our actions to ourselves, we add lying to the mix.

The yogi sees that there is an abundance in the world, not a lack, and that to take something that is not freely given shows an imbalance, a distortion of the human personality. Because he has no desires and feels no envy, he is content with what he has and counts on his Self to provide him with everything he will need, at just the right time. Because he lives in abundance he is able to give freely and unconditionally of everything he has, and the world rewards him in return.

Sexual moderation means celibacy to a monk, and the release and transformation of sexual energy into the spiritual life can lead to a heightened spirituality. The yogis, like the Taoists, believe that sexual energy is a potent form of life energy, and that ejaculation drains away this life force. To conserve this energy we need to be sexually moderate.

For people who reject celibacy and believe that sexuality should be another form of spirituality, sexual moderation means acting without exploitation of others, not using other people's bodies for one's own gratification. In a sexual relationship, we interchange our deepest creative energies with another person, and join our two selves in a physical and spiritual unity. This mingling of two selves, two sexual energies, if treated lovingly, openly and reverentially, can regenerate our spirituality and deepen our commitment. This is much more than just the friction of two bodies to release built-up tension.

But to get to this state means being willing to open your-self to your partner's deepest truth, and to allow your truth to be equally open and transparent. Complete trust is required, and an unconditional giving of Self.

We only know ourselves when we are in a relationship with another person, when we see our attitudes and behaviour reflected back at us. This knowledge is the most important learning experience we can have.

If we are in a permanent relationship, it means remaining faithful in the face of temptation, even though this is often difficult. This ties into non-lying; if I decide to sleep with someone and only I know it, what harm can there be? My partner will never know, and what she doesn't know can't harm her. But lying to yourself like this is a kind of silent poisoning which over time destroys the relationship from within. The truth invariably seeps out, since the lie still exists in our unconscious, and the guilt we feel makes certain that it will be revealed at the worst possible time.

The singles scene is also closely tied in to deception and lying. It's easy to flit from one relationship to another, taking off when the possibility of commitment arises, leaving confusion, pain and broken hearts behind.

Non-greed, non-possessiveness points out what all five of these teachings are aiming at. We are greedy because we are scared and insecure, and we use money and possessions to shore up our weak sense of Self. All five of the yamas relate to our selfish ego and the need we feel to keep it secure by giving it sustenance. In my fear I cling to myself, act only for myself, consider myself first, and identify my small self with objects – my money, status and possessions. I feel separate, alienated and isolated from others, and in that isolation I act selfishly.

The yogi trusts in his Self, in God and in the universe (which to him are just different names for the same thing) to sustain him and provide for him. His security is not provided by his attachment to things or people, but by the oneness that he feels about all life, and the abundance of life itself. This is his freedom, an abiding awareness of his own inner source, and a knowledge that what is essential is already with him. He has no need to seek happiness in outside things; happiness is already there, just waiting to be discovered.

The Niyamas / Personal Observance

Purity is a word we don't use any more because it sounds too holy and sanctimonious, and publicly we don't make distinctions between pure and impure. But privately I believe we do, and this relates especially to personal health. One of the reasons I don't smoke is because I don't want my lungs to become black and stiff like tarpaper. I'd rather keep them pink and healthy, functioning well, and if this means keeping them 'pure', then so be it.

To have a healthy body requires an element of purity, in that you don't want to pollute what used to be called 'your temple'. Our concern with organic food and clean drinking water, the pollution of the environment and the treatment of animals, are all important concerns that relate to purity in a non-sanctimonious way. If we want a healthy world, we need to start by cultivating a healthy mind and body, stable, harmonious, balanced and pure. The reason we do this is not only because we want to lead a longer, healthier life, but also because we respect life itself, in the form of our body, mind and spirit, and in doing this we extend our respect to the earth, which is our mother.

Contentment and tranquillity are the Holy Grail of the spiritual path. We can achieve this state of calm and stillness when we manage to let go of our limited selfish desires and instead find a healthier relationship with the world, one in which we discover our true Self and identify with others. To do this, we need to place our trust in something greater than ourselves, and rely on that unknown something to provide us with the sustenance we require.

We need to find a way fully to accept not just who we are and where life has taken us, but to move on from that point with a fearlessness and a willingness to accept whatever happens in the future. If we enter the future in league with others and work for the benefit of all, then the fear and insecurity that destroy contentment and tranquillity can be eliminated. As the *Bhagavad Gita* says,

> *A person who has been able to let go of all personal desires and is completely content in the truth of his Self, is someone whose soul has found peace. A person whose mind is not troubled by sorrows and has no longing for pleasure and happiness, who is beyond passion, fear and anger – that is someone of steady wisdom. One who is free of all mental attachments and neither rejoices when good things happen nor feels repelled when bad happens, maintains a serene wisdom.*

Discipline is another word that we prefer not to use any more, but it is impossible to move forward in yoga without it. It takes discipline to turn up week after week for a yoga class, discipline to find the time to practise or meditate at home, discipline to follow spiritual teachings in a consumer society that considers them old-fashioned and irrelevant. Without discipline, most people give up on themselves, and live to regret it.

Discipline also means the willingness to give up something of ourselves, an act of self-sacrifice that provides a control over sensual desires, rather than always being a victim to those desires. We need to accept that we can't get everything we want or do everything we desire, and so discipline means that our selfish ego becomes reduced, and we become open to a larger view of life. This expansion of consciousness enables us to make better decisions about things, learning to discriminate between the essential and the superfluous. To do this shows a certain maturity and means that we are able to grow beyond our childhood illusions.

The *Yoga Sutras* say that Nature is the great teacher of the Self. Nature provides us with experiences that we decide are 'good' or 'bad', and it is through these experiences, particularly the ones that provide us with pain and loss, that we learn about ourselves. This school of hard knocks is the great teacher, for as Lancelot Law Whyte has said, 'Thought is born of failure.' It is only when we have been disappointed and defeated that we realize the need to change our attitudes and responses to life, and through coping with experiences of failure are able to grow and extend ourselves into something greater and finer.

Study means thinking and reflecting about life and its meaning, and most important of all, it means studying yourself: your body, thoughts, feelings, memories and Spirit. It means acquiring self-knowledge through meditation and reflection.

It also means reading books that encourage spiritual values, no matter whether these are scriptures, novels or poetry. Wisdom is available from those who have trail-blazed for us, and we can use their guidance in exploring our own path. But the ultimate answer we seek is not in books, but in ourselves.

Devotion is the third term of the niyamas that we no longer use. What Patanjali means here is devotion to God, but it is not devotion to a creator God like the Jewish YHWH or to the eternal and all-powerful Hindu God, the Divine principle

Brahman. Patanjali has in mind devotion or respect to a personal God, a God who is more knowledgeable and powerful than we are and whom we individually look up to. This God represents whatever ideals we personally hold most important and attempt to emulate.

The Self within, our true ruler and the source of all our knowledge, is effectively this personal God, since it represents the truth of our being, the truth of ourselves that we hold in the heart and express through every cell of our body. When we live by this truth, we are God-like, and we really have found God. Devotion consists in loving this Self and in devoting all our actions selflessly to it, not taking personal credit for these actions and not expecting any beneficial rewards from them. This devotion and love give a massive sense of security and courage, while denying this truth, and trying to live only for our own benefit, leads to fear, insecurity and alienation.

Patanjali believes that all ten of these ethical teachings form a critical part of yoga training and need to be practised both inside and outside the yoga hall if we are to make any spiritual progress in life. Our contemporary culture is quite sceptical about practising things called discipline and purity, since anything that smacks of self-restraint is to be avoided. We live in a selfish society that does not want to admit any restraint on desire. Desire is what keeps us shopping, and is the basis of our entire social and commercial system. But if we understand that the practice of discipline and purity is beneficial and actually makes us feel better, both physically and mentally, we can learn to swim against the tide of public opinion and gain some true independence for ourselves.

8

Physical Training: Asanas

The ancient texts say that there are potentially 184,000 asanas or positions that the body can take, but in normal practice there are usually considered to be eighty-four, of which about thirty are used today. There are many fine books on yoga which detail the positions and how to get into them properly, but practice should preferably start with a qualified teacher, since it is not recommended (and nearly impossible) to teach yourself yoga properly.

The type of yoga that has captured the interest of the West is called Hatha Yoga and its popularity is due to its focus on the postures of the body, the asanas. The popular image of yoga is of someone, usually a young and svelte woman, holding a graceful asana position and looking positively beatific. Yoga has become fashionable, and its image has consequently become intertwined with contemporary images that relate to mainstream fashion – idealizations of attractiveness and beauty.

This concern for a specific body look has led many women into yoga, where they hope that diligent practice will trim and tone their body to the required shape. I don't have to point out how far removed a body-based yoga practice like this is from the spiritual ideal proposed by Patanjali, and this is surely a case of missing the goal by concentrating on the technique. The ultimate goal is freedom, but who is less free than a person trapped by the dictates of a fashion designer, or whose entire will-power is turned towards the achievement of a fashion editor's ideal of beauty?

This book attempts to put the practice of yoga into a larger context, in which daily or weekly practice can be located as part of a systematic philosophy whose ultimate aim is the total liberation of the human spirit, allowing a spontaneous flowering of the immense potential locked away in all of us. How can I make the connection between the absolute heaven of this spiritual dimension, and the sweaty polished wood floor where so many people are happy to settle for so much less, and are probably unaware of how much more yoga is able to offer? What is the difference between the attitude and behaviour of a yogi on the yoga mat and that of a body-oriented practitioner?

In an advanced and ideal state, the yogi no longer identifies her Self with her body or her mind, but identifies only with her Spirit, her inner Self. She very likely didn't always hold this attitude, but discovered it through a long and diligent practice of yoga, a living philosophy.

Her aim in doing the asanas is not only to increase flexibility, fitness and strength, but primarily to release tension held in her body, to loosen it, soften it, open it, so that internal blockages and obstructions, formed by old negative emotions and thoughts, can be shaken up, cleansed and washed away, allowing the body's internal pathways and organs to become clear. In this open state her living energy, her prana, can be free-flowing and move unhindered through her body. This is a true state of health.

The yogi achieves this openness by performing her asanas mindfully, working gently with her body and not forcing it into 'perfect' positions. To work with the body means using the breath to extend and elongate naturally, and to use the force of gravity to root the heaviness of the lower body to the earth, allowing the light upper body to float upwards to the sky. Breathing relaxes the spine and muscles and allows the body to grow and release tension. Since periods of growth are not continuous, the yogi willingly contrasts periods of movement with periods of rest, respecting her body, so that its natural intelligence can consolidate what it has attained.

To work mindfully means to focus awareness on the movement and the breath acting together, so that such single-pointed concentration unites the body, breath and mind into the present moment – the now, this instant – the living breathing moment in which the yogi is aware of that everyday miracle – her life.

Acting like this, focusing her awareness on what really matters, there is no need, and certainly no desire, to cast glances around the room to see how others are doing, or to worry about whether her pose is 'perfect' according to some guru's rule-book. That kind of ambitious, competitive, external, goal-oriented, attached thinking is not where yoga is at.

Intensely alive in the moment, aware of the breath travelling in and out that is her primary source of life, feeling her living, pulsating body supported fully by the generous earth, the yogi's openness permeates her entire body, reaching her heart and allowing it to open, thereby radiating throughout the entire universe the hidden treasures of tenderness, love and compassion that she stores in her inmost heart. These treasures are not hers alone, but have been given to her as blessings from God, to share with all. She feels that the goodness, compassion and love that she holds are really God's qualities, unconditionally offered at all times.

We all share these tender feelings, but most of us hide our treasures out of fear, to protect ourselves from imagined pain. This is why, in our world, they have become so rare.

The *Bhagavad Gita* says of life;

The sages say that whoever does things without personal desire
for success is wise. That person's actions are pure and he knows

the truth. In whatever work he does, such a person has peace: he expects nothing, and he relies on nothing. He does nothing, although he is always engaged in action. Having given up desire, with control over his mind and ego, he is free from all attachments, and only his body works.

He is free from sin. He is happy with whatever the universe has given to him and is not attached to pleasure or pain; he is happy whether he succeeds or not and is not bound by his actions.

When you let go of all attachments and experience liberation, you find peace in wisdom.

If everyone who practised yoga would take this attitude into the yoga hall, and learn to keep and maintain it outside in 'real life', they would soon find themselves living in a much kinder, more thoughtful, more positive and more loving world, one in which they could find that peace in wisdom. And your world too would instantly begin to transform the moment you made such an attitude your own.

9

Breath Control – Pranayama

Although Hatha Yoga has developed an elaborate asana system for bodily strength, its primary focus is on the prana, the life energy, which is worked on by a system of purifying breathing exercises called pranayama.

The word Hatha is derived from *ha*, meaning sun, and *tha*, meaning moon, which is in itself a reference to pranayama. *Ha* is the positive right nostril representing the sun and *tha* is the negative left nostril representing the moon. Hatha practice is intended to bring both sides into balance to keep our nature in equilibrium. Hatha work also includes meditation, chanting OM and other mantras, and other internal cleansing practices.

Hatha Yoga was developed quite late in yoga terms, in the ninth to tenth centuries CE in Nepal, by the Nath yogis Matsyendra and Goraksa. They were interested both in cultivating strength of body and in developing martial arts. This interest in physical strength is still a feature of Nepal, as shown by the bravery and physical endurance of the Gurkhas and Sherpas of that region.

The Nath yogis used the regulation of breath in order to gain increasing control over their unconscious functions. The muscle that makes the link between asanas and pranayama is the diaphragm, which we can either consciously control or unconsciously allow the brain to operate. This link between the conscious and the unconscious was developed by the Nath yogis in order to acquire special psychic powers called siddhas. These include the ability to move among people without being seen, the ability to project oneself on others' attention, the ability to levitate or alternatively to stay motionless, to become omniscient, and to suspend all physical activities. These powers include the famous ability of yogis to stay buried alive for long periods of time (see the story of Haridas in Chapter 2).

The Nath yogis' system of pranayama was intended to release the intense energy that is usually trapped in our bodies, specifically at the base of the spine. This energy, called kundalini, and visualized as a coiled serpent sitting immobile at the bottom of the spine, is woken by specific breathing practices. Once it is aroused, the yogi directs this energy into a central channel, or as acupuncturists would say a meridian, which runs all the way up the spine to the skull. Along the way, the kundalini energy opens and vitalizes the six chakras (wheels) which are energy nodes located inside the body.

The *Yoga Sutras* consider these special powers as an entertaining (and potentially dangerous) side-show and not the main aim of yoga, but it is important that we learn to regulate our breath in order to maximize our health, both physical and spiritual. Every ancient society that evolved a 'teaching' or a philosophy of life considered the breath as one of the keys to life. In Greece there was the pneuma, in China the chi, and in India the prana. The Hebrew Bible emphasized the importance of breath, when Adam was brought to life by God, in Genesis 2:9:

And YHWH, God, formed the human of dust from the soil, and he blew into his nostrils the breath of life and the human became a living being.

Arthur Waskow has pointed out that if you try to say aloud the name of God, YHWH, you realize that all you are doing is forming a loud breath. The ancients always thought in an associated way, which compared like to like, so wind and breath were seen as comprising a similar element: the air in the atmosphere and the breath in our bodies were the same thing.

People knew that a person could survive for quite a few days without food and water, but without breath life ceases in minutes. Consequently breath was considered the first element of life, and its use in training the mind and body was identified very early on.

There is a Chan (Chinese Zen) story that illuminates both this dependence on breath and the habitual ease with which we fall into the habit of taking our life energy for granted:

A young monk was meditating by following his breath, as he had been taught by his Master. After days of meditating like this he complained that it was boring just to follow his breath. Wasn't there some other practice to follow?

The Master considered the question and walked the young monk over to a full barrel of water. Without warning, he pushed the monk's head into the water and held it submerged for thirty seconds before releasing him.

The monk emerged gasping for breath, and the Master said, 'Still bored with following your breath?'

Breathing is used as a practice and a discipline in the East because it provides a vital link between the somatic and the autonomic nervous systems. If you do not attempt to control your breath, your primitive brain stem will automatically 'breathe' you unconsciously through the autonomic nervous system. Your primitive brain is programmed to breathe you all through your life. However, we have the ability to deliberately channel and regulate the breath through our conscious mind, and when we do this we create a bridge between the two nervous systems, and hence between our conscious and unconscious minds.

Since mental health is a function of the maximum use of the unconscious mind or a complete integration of the conscious and the unconscious, the practice of breath control is a way to increase the overall well-being of the individual.

When we breathe badly we create obstructions in various parts of our body. All these blockages clog up the full free flow of prana, the life breath that animates our body. Through practices like pranayama we learn how to move and generate prana, to store it and to use it. We are then able to loosen and dissolve these obstructions so that the prana can flow freely, giving us the freedom that we once enjoyed as very young children, but which we lost with increasing education, exclusive dependence on rational thinking, and poor use of the mind.

In yoga we invite the breath into the body, and by inhaling we invite the entire energy of the universe to enter us and fill us. When exhaling we remove whatever toxins and impurities have collected in us, and we feel able to let go and undo, while the body relaxes. Yoga training is basic, fundamental and a grounding for life. It teaches us that by working consciously with the breath, we can gain a small intimation of the incredible control and discipline that advanced yogis can accomplish with their bodies, able to cease breathing for hours at a time, able consciously to control their heartbeat, their body temperature and other bodily functions that to us are only operated unconsciously.

Since the body, breath and mind are all interconnected, we cannot move a muscle without first having moved our mind in terms of the intention to make that move, and we also breathe whenever we initiate a physical movement. The combination of using the mind to direct our muscles in a specific way, and using our breath to help us make that move smooth and graceful, means that even in the most physical part of yoga we are starting to train our entire organism to become single-minded, directed in purpose. This single-mindedness is carried through from asanas to pranayama (breath control), and then into meditation, with each rung of the yoga ladder directing the mind further inward and focusing the mind one-pointedly into greater concentration.

We begin to understand how a greater conscious control over ourselves can be attempted, and no matter how small a change this makes (most of us do not seek to be miracle workers), we gain confidence that we are able to effect some conscious control over ourselves and do not have to go through life either as slaves to old ingrained habits or as automatons of our unconscious impulses. Yoga, by increasing self-confidence in our practice, enables us to extend this confidence into other areas of our life – work, parenting, social life, sexuality, sport and play.

IO

Meditation

In asana we work mostly on the gross physical body, and in pranayama we move inwards, working chiefly with the more subtle breath. The next move is still further inwards and towards even more subtlety as we begin to work directly with the mind. The breath has now become quiet and still, and the mind has become more settled. Patanjali lists the four meditational states individually:

Pratyahara	Withdrawing the senses
Dharana	Concentration
Dhayana	Meditation
Samadhi	Absorption

However, it is clear that these are really linked states of consciousness, whereby one moves imperceptibly from one to the next. The boundaries between these states of being are not really firmly delineated but are fluid and permeable. Nor are they linear in one direction, and it is quite possible to go back from one stage to another, instead of always going forwards.

By moving our attention inwards, we automatically withdraw our senses from the outer world, since we are no longer concerned with exercising the physical body or controlling the breath. The eyes are no longer looking out at the objects of the world, the ears are not straining to listen, the body is held immobile, the breath becomes quiet and under control, and it is the mind that now becomes the object of concentration. With eyes either partially or completely closed, we now begin to meditate, which to the ancient yogis was the heart of yoga. When we meditate regularly, a peaceful, quiet, contented feeling comes over body and mind. The body settles down to a homeostasis, and eventually the mind settles.

The problem everyone has with meditation is the difficulty of stilling the mind, of stopping the thoughts that continually race and whirl around it. This is the very heart of Patanjali's system:

Yoga means to still the swirling currents of thoughts in the mind. If you can control the thoughts that arise, and still them completely, you are able to observe the world clearly and directly without the distortions of the ego. The ability to discipline the chattering mind is what takes us to the state of yoga.

When the turbulence stops and the lake of the mind becomes clear and still, our true essence, our Self or Spirit, is reflected. Then the Self can abide in its own true nature. This is the goal, this is what we want to attain.

When we fail to still our minds we mistakenly identify our Self with the activities of the mind, and become lost in our thoughts. We lose the true sense of who we are because we have lost sight of our true essence, our real inner Self.

Unless we can still these thoughts, we are unable to hear the silence behind them, which is our background awareness and in which we can discover the open freedom that yoga promises us: the pure awareness that is our existence and our joy. In this samadhi or absorption – a feeling of great clarity, openness, adaptability and freedom – we discover our true being, which is in fact our unique, unspoken truth. Our aim, and it is not easy, is to extend this feeling and bring our unique truth with us when we emerge from meditation into everyday life, so that we begin to alter the way we use our body, the way we breathe and the way we use our mind. We need to find a way to maintain the truthful awareness of our inner Self and not have it immediately swamped and covered again by our limited ego's fears and insecurities.

The great Zen Buddhist Thich Nhat Hanh says that it helps to meditate on the image of a pebble thrown into a river. How is one helped by the image of a pebble? Sit down in whatever position suits you best, the Half Lotus or Lotus, or even in a straight-backed chair, and keep a half-smile on your face.

Breathe slowly and deeply, following each breath, becoming one with each breath. Then let go of everything. Imagine yourself as a pebble that has been thrown into a river. The pebble sinks through the water effortlessly; detached from everything, it falls by the shortest distance possible, finally sinking to the bottom, the point of perfect rest. You are like a pebble that has let itself fall into the river, letting go of everything. At the centre of your being is your breath. You don't need to know the length of time it takes to reach the point of complete rest on the bed of fine sand beneath the water. But when you feel yourself resting like a pebble that has settled on the riverbed, that is the point when you begin to find your own rest, your own peace. In that peace you are no longer pushed or pulled by anything.

I have an image that I use to convey the sense of emptying my mind of thoughts. From a vantage-point high above, I picture myself sitting in meditation on the floor of the main hall of a huge deserted main-line railway station. I am completely alone, my eyes shut, the empty floor spreading out in all directions, and there is a muffled, almost underwater silence in this entire vast space.

Trains, like trains of thought, are at every moment silently gliding out from dozens of platforms to all possible destinations, and these trains represent all the thoughts, memories, feelings, desires, fears, ruminations, reflections, speculations, words, tunes and images that bombard me when I first sit down to meditate. But I, settling down into a deep and peaceful meditative state, stay seated in the terminus, do not feel tempted to board any of these trains, and will not pursue the connections that they inevitably go on to make, thought endlessly leading on to thought. I avoid these trains of thought by staying in the pure awareness of this hall, happy to remain in solitary and silent contemplation of my own awareness, itself an immense cavernous void like the station, where I am rapt in the infinite stillness of eternity.

This infinite stillness is bliss, and the only heaven I am likely to experience. But what a heaven!

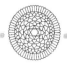

II

The Origins of Yoga

The early history of yoga lies buried with the dust and bricks of past civilizations, and there is no way that we can unearth its true origins. But the West has had contact with Indian civilization for over 2,300 years, and these varying encounters brought practising yogis into view of the Western mind. In this chapter I will detail some of these encounters, and explain how in the eighteenth and nineteenth centuries the British attempted to discover and understand the Hindu culture from which yoga emerged. The British involvement in India led to an evolutionary reform of Indian culture and religion that brought the first influential yogi to the West in 1893. That first contact, at the very end of the nineteenth century, has blossomed into the 20 million or more yoga students who currently practise in Western countries.

Classical Encounters

The West first became aware of yogis in classical times, when Alexander the Great invaded the Punjab in 326 BCE. In India Alexander discovered advanced civilizations, powerful armies, and a strong philosophical and religious culture, with influential holy men or yogis. The Greeks called these yogis 'gymnosophists', meaning naked philosophers, because the

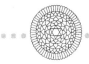

ones they met were 'sky-clad' monks who had renounced everything, including clothes. Plutarch, in his *Life of Alexander*, supposedly recorded what was known of Alexander's discussions with these holy men:

Once he captured ten gymnosophists, who were reputed to have the ability to answer questions cleverly and pithily, so Alexander put a series of questions to them, with the warning that he would kill the first one who gave a wrong answer, and then the rest, one after another, on the same principle. He started with the eldest, and asked him whether the living or the dead were more numerous: 'The living,' the yogi said, 'because the dead no longer exist.' The fifth was asked which came first, day or night, and he replied, 'Day, by a day.' Alexander looked puzzled at this answer, so the gymnosophist said that hard questions were bound to have hard answers.

Alexander moved to the sixth holy man and asked him how a man could best win popularity: 'By being extremely powerful,' he said, 'without being an object of fear.' Another was asked how a man might become a god: 'By doing something,' he answered, 'that a man cannot do.' The next one was asked which was stronger, life or death: 'Life,' he said, 'because it carries so much suffering.' And the last one was asked how long a man should live: 'Until he has stopped considering death preferable to life,' he replied.

Alexander later met a yogi whose fame lasted for hundreds of years because of his unflinching attitude towards death. His name was said to be Sphines, but since he greeted everyone with the Indian word '*kali*', the Greeks called him Calanus. He was the only yogi who agreed to accompany Alexander and his army on their return West, but in Persia he became seriously ill, suffering from a stomach disorder. He asked for a funeral pyre to be built, and, after being carried to the pyre on horseback, he offered up a prayer to the gods, purified himself with a sprinkling of water, and consecrated some of his hair. Now ready, he climbed the pyre, greeted the Greeks who were there, and prophesied that he would soon be seeing the king in Babylon. Then he lay down, covered his head, and the pyre was lit. The Greeks were astonished that the approaching flames did not make him flinch or cry out, and Calanus stayed in exactly the same spot without moving, making an acceptable sacrifice of himself in accordance with his tradition.

Three hundred years later, Apollonius of Tyana, a wizard, philosopher, healer and mystic who lived during the first century CE, made a trip to India expressly to meet the Indian holy men, who he believed were wiser and more godly than their equivalents in the Roman world. Meeting the leader of a group of yogis, Apollonius supposedly asked if they knew themselves, expecting them to be like the Greeks in thinking it difficult to know oneself. But the yogi surprised him by saying, 'We know everything because we begin by knowing ourselves. None of us would approach our kind of philosophy without knowing himself first.'

Apollonius then asked what they thought they were, and the yogi replied, 'Gods.' 'Why?' asked Apollonius. 'Because we are good men.' Apollonius thought this an enlightened view, and he went on to ask their belief about the soul. 'It is what Pythagoras taught you Greeks and we taught the Egyptians,' answered the yogi, meaning that the soul or Self is eternal and lives on after death, reincarnating into another body. This teaching formed part of Plato's beliefs, and it is likely that he learned it from followers of Pythagoras. It seems very possible that Pythagoras in turn was influenced by Indian ideas.

Whether Alexander or Apollonius actually had these exact conversations with yogis is highly unlikely, but it is clear that the yogis made a very strong impression on them, an impression that was to repeat itself 2,100 years later.

The British Discover the Aryans

Once the Western Roman Empire fell in the fifth century CE, meetings between East and West were largely curtailed for over 1,000 years, until empire-building Europeans began once again to venture East. In the seventeenth century, the British began to seek trade and power in India, and Clive's military defeat of the Nawab of Bengal in 1757 led to the long British Raj, or reign. For the next 200 years the British ruled India as a colony, part of its widespread Empire.

The attitude of the largely Eurocentric and racist British officers towards India was similar to their view of Africa, which they regarded as a place of more or less decadent savages who had repellent customs, no civilization or culture to speak of, and whose Hindu religion was a disgusting polytheistic heathen mixture of cow and monkey worship and bloodthirsty and many-limbed gods. The uptight and sexually repressed British were shocked at the Indians' easy-going attitude to nudity and eroticism, as John Marshall, a factor of the East India Company, was to report:

> *Some yogis go stark naked, several of which I have seen in India, and 'tis reported that the Hindu women will go to them and kiss the yogi's yard. Others lay something upon it when it stands, which the yogis take to buy victuals with; and several come to stroke it, thinking that there is a good deal of virtue in it, none having gone out of it, as they say, for they lie not with women nor use any other way to vent their seed.*

By the end of the eighteenth century, British historians could trace Indian history back to the time of the Muslim invasions and conquest, around 1000 CE, but working back from this time to Alexander's incursion of 326 BCE, some 1,300 years, they had a total blank about India during this period. The Indians themselves believed their civilization was an ancient one, but had no written histories or chronicles to prove this, other than undated lists of kings and emperors. There seemed to be no way of discovering what occurred in this vast country during the 1,300-year-long void. The story of the unveiling of this history, and the discovery of an ancient civilization predating Alexander by a further 2,000 years, is one of the most intriguing by-products of the 200-year-long British Raj.

It was the ancient sacred language of Sanskrit that held the first key to the mystery. The origins of Sanskrit were unknown, and it was virtually a dead language, spoken by very few people and used mainly by the Brahmins, the Hindu priests, in their religious rituals. All the most ancient religious writings, the *Vedas* (a word meaning knowledge or revealed truth) were composed in Sanskrit, but the dates of these scriptures were also unknown. The idea arose that there might be clues in these writings that could contribute to the search for India's lost history.

In 1785 a British printer named Charles Wilkins made the first translation from Sanskrit into English when he published a version of the *Bhagavad Gita, The Celestial Song*. This work, the best-loved and most influential of all Indian scriptures, had a disarming effect on the Empire builders. Rather than emphasizing a polytheistic creed, the *Bhagavad Gita* portrayed a single loving god in the form of Krishna, who declared an ethical philosophy that was worthy of the highest of Christian ideals. This scripture forced the more narrow-minded British to revise their opinion of Hinduism and to take seriously the Indian claim to a culture that appeared to be even older than their own. From looking on the Indians as 'creatures scarce above the degree of savage life', they now had to consider that they were in fact heirs to an ancient and remarkable civilization. The subject of Indian studies gained respectability.

In 1784 Sir William Jones, a polymath scholar and

Supreme Court Judge in Calcutta, learned Bengali and Sanskrit and was surprised to discover that the Indian mind had invented, among other things, chess, algebra, trigonometry, the Western number system (including the all-important zero) and the pentatonic scale in music, as well as having devised a complete medical practice, the Ayurvedic, and a fully developed legal, ethical and philosophical system – and all this before the earliest Greek thinkers.

Jones made a particular study of Sanskrit language and grammar and was surprised to find striking resemblances to Greek and Latin. For example, the Sanskrit word for mother was *matr*, and that for mouse *mus*. These similarities were too numerous to be merely the result of chance, so Jones devised a theory that these languages, together with Germanic, Celtic and Old Persian, had all derived from a common source, a language that was no longer extant. He called this theoretical common-source language Aryan; later called 'Indo-European', it gave its name to the large family of languages that spread from Western Europe to India. What was radical about Jones's theory was that in showing that all these languages came from a single source it demonstrated a common ethnicity between the British rulers and their Northern Indian subjects, which must have made some of the Empire builders uncomfortable.

With the new detailed knowledge of Sanskrit, it now became possible to compare the syllables, words and grammar of the Vedic scriptures and examine the changes that took place in the language over time. By this means it became possible to determine which texts were early and which late. Although an inexact science, this meant that an approximate time-scale could be made for the scriptures, which could help to determine a rough Indian historical chronology.

The oldest *Veda*, the *Rig Veda*, a collection of religious hymns, was dated to about 1100 BCE, making it the world's oldest known written scripture. It was clear that these hymns were far more ancient than even this date, since they had been transmitted orally for generations before being written down. From the evidence in the different *Vedas*, British and other European scholars built up a picture of the people who composed these hymns. Because of the similarity between Sanskrit and the Iranian group of languages they assumed that the people who described themselves as Arya were invaders of India, not indigenous to the land. The Arya had a technological superiority over the local people in the form of iron tools and horse-drawn chariots, and they were pictured as combative warriors who defeated the indigenous tribes, appropriated their livestock and became rulers of India. Their reign was assumed to be from 1500 BCE to 500 BCE.

The Arya were presumed to be nomadic pastoralists rather than farmers or city-dwellers. They roamed with their herds and performed elaborate animal and plant sacrifices to their gods, who were often personifications of nature and the elements, similar to the Greek gods. The Arya were outgoing, nature-loving, life-affirming materialists, and they were seen as fine-featured, tall, fair-skinned and superior people. In contrast, the indigenous people, the Dasa or Dasyu, were characterized as dark-skinned, small, flatnosed, uncouth, backward and inferior. This scholarly racism reflected many of the European prejudices about India, as John Keay, in *A History of India*, describes:

> *Nineteenth-century British colonists, reflecting on this new and unexpected Aryan dimension to India's history, could draw great comfort. All that was fine and 'classical' in ancient India's history could now be credited to this influx of manly heroes from the West. The Aryans, spreading their superior culture right down the valley of the Ganga and then deep into*

the peninsula, had conferred on India an unprecedented cultural integrity and an enviably high degree of civilization. In time, however, the purity of the Aryan race had become hopelessly diluted; manliness, creativity and drive had succumbed to the enervating effects of an intolerable climate and an insidious social system . . . India had slumped into seemingly irredeemable decadence and degeneracy. Then, in the nick of time, out of the West came the British. No less fair, no less manly and no less confident of their superiority, they were the neo-Aryans, galvanizing a naturally lax people into endeavour and industry, showering them with the incomparable benefits of a superior civilization and a humane religion, and ushering in a new and golden age.

The dark side of this racialist concept became obvious in the 1930s when the Nazis decided that they were the true inheritors of Aryan culture, the master race of pure Nordic blood, who were destined to rule over all non-Aryans, in particular the Semitic Jews. The consequent oppression of all non-Aryans led to cruelty, genocide and inhumanity on a scale undreamt of till then. Aryanization proved to be brutality and barbarism.

At the same time, archaeologists in India were making findings that would push the pre-history of Indian civilization back a further 2,000 years and would call into question the nature of the Arya. Sometime in the late 1860s, a British officer, Major Clark, had been doing some amateur excavating in extensive brick ruins at Harappa, on the Ravi river in the Punjab, when he came across a small seal buried there. The seal was made of a smooth, unpolished black stone and featured a bull and some letters that no one could decipher.

It was in 1921 that a proper excavation of the site took place, and more seals and pottery were found. But the breakthrough did not occur until 1922 when an Indian archaeologist, R. D. Banerji, excavated a site called Mohenjo-daro, where there were extensive ruins around a Buddhist stupa and monastery. Here Banerji discovered four layers of strata under the stupa, the earliest being of the second century CE. This meant that the oldest had to be very old indeed, and when Banerji found more of the seals with the strange pictograph writing, he knew that the sites of Harappa and Mohenjo-daro were of the same civilization and the same age.

This new 'cradle of civilization' became known as the Indus Valley Civilization, and it brought Indian pre-history back by at least 1,500 years before the Arya culture, down to 3500–3000 BCE. The two sites were excavated properly and later more examples of the Indus Valley culture were found spread throughout India. The sites were all planned towns built out of a standardized size of brick, with roomy houses fitted with wells and drainage systems, and mathematically regulated road widths. The regularity of the technology, which had remained unaltered for 1,000 years, came as a great surprise to the archaeologists. But what was of greater surprise to yoga scholars was one of the seals found in Mohenjo-daro.

This seal showed a figure seated in a cross-legged yogic asana posture. The figure either has enormous horns or is wearing a headdress, and its long, serious face could either be a mask or three faces looking in different directions. The figure also either has an erect penis or is wearing something hanging from a belt buckle. Around the seated figure stand various animals, and beneath the low stool are two deer. This figure has been recognized as a possible prototype of the god Siva, who was always considered the ideal yogi and Lord of the Beasts. What is important about the seal is that the cross-legged posture shows that as long ago as 3500 BCE a form of yoga was already known and practised in India, and that it predated the Hindu religion, which is an outgrowth of the Aryan *Vedas*.

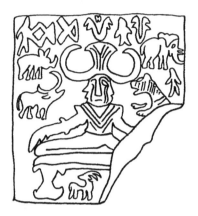

The 'yoga-seal' from the Indus Valley

The contrast between the Aryan and Indus Valley cultures is great. The Arya people had a priesthood which memorized and preserved voluminous prayers, but preserved no buildings or artefacts, whilst the Indus Valley people were the first highly organized town planners who left numerous cities but no sign of a religion, and an as yet undeciphered pictographic script. If I were to speculate as to which society might have generated the first yogis, my vote would be with the Indus Valley, for two reasons.

First, the seal is a strong piece of evidence that yogic practices were known, recognized and accepted by the Indus Valley people. Second, when the Arya sacrificed to their gods, they drank a nectar called soma, which was derived from a yellow plant found in the mountains. Soma, which they also considered divine, identifying it with Indra, the warrior god, was clearly an intoxicant intended to provide an altered state of consciousness, an ecstatic state during the ceremony. In street terms, the Arya were high as kites when they sacrificed to their gods, and they used this state of intoxication to become fearless and strong in battle.

Since classical yoga provides a natural high, a spiritual absorption in samadhi with no need for drugs or intoxicants, it seems to me that the two are mutually exclusive. It is impossible to practise yogic concentration and meditation under the influence of drink or drugs, although with drugs it is clearly possible to reach other states of spiritual ecstasy. Mircea Eliade, in his book *Yoga, Immortality and Freedom*, makes the point that drugs other than soma were used by ascetics during the Rig Veda period, and that yogis seeking special magical powers also made use of them. Swami Satchidananda, who arrived in America in the 1960s and was taken up by the first generation to experiment with drugs on a large scale, said of his young druggy followers:

> *Drugs give a brought-in experience, not developed by one's own Self. It's not a genuine spiritual experience. It is something like a medicinally-induced sleep. They said they wanted to expand their consciousness. But when the drugs failed them they turned to yoga consciousness. As they continued the purifying yoga practice, their use of drugs simply fell away naturally.*

To rely on drugs to acquire a state of ecstasy or mental power is clearly to be attached, and shows a pronounced non-yogic clinging to desire.

No one knows why the Indus Valley civilization came to an end, but it seems safe to assume that the yogic practices developed there were practised, refined and embodied by yogis who managed to live on after its fall. As they mingled with the mélange of other tribes and races, their yogic ideas came to be incorporated over time by the descendants of the Arya people, who merged the Indus Valley form of yoga with their own ascetic practices. In this way a synthesized form of yoga became a central feature of Hinduism, which has always allowed a wide acceptance of different beliefs and practices under its roof.

When Jainism and Buddhism broke off from Hinduism, around the fifth century BCE, yoga remained as an essential mainstay of these new spiritual endeavours. The Buddha is perhaps the best-known of all yogis, and his enlightenment while sitting under the banyan tree in Boddh Gaya is an example of the power of yogic meditation. Through Buddhism, yoga became a widespread practice, travelling with the new religion to China, Japan, Tibet, Ceylon, Thailand, Mongolia, Burma and so on.

How Yoga Came West

The introduction of Christianity to India by British missionaries forced Hinduism to reform its practices, in particular the sacrifice of animals, grotesque child marriage, temple prostitution, the burning of widows, the stultifying caste system and untouchability. These attempts to reform ancient religious and social mores encouraged a spiritual renewal which regenerated Hinduism. In the nineteenth century a number of reformist movements evolved, and the one of most importance for Western yoga was based around Ramakrishna Paramahamsa.

I am going to spend some time detailing the character and influence of Sri Ramakrishna and his relationship with his disciple Swami Vivekananda, because Vivekananda was the first yogi to make a major impact in the West. Since these two men effectively represent the first source of yoga teaching in America, I think it would be helpful to understand the religious and spiritual background that spawned them.

Their relationship of guru and disciple is intense and unique, and reveals much about how yoga is thought of in India and how it is taught. These men were yogis, but they didn't seem to spend very much time in asanas, other than the Lotus posture for meditation. Instead, they each followed their own spiritual path, which for Ramakrishna was a form of Bhakti Yoga, in which whole-hearted devotion to God, here represented by the goddess Kali, the Mother, was his form of unification. Ramakrishna hungered for God with a tremendous passion, and he wanted a complete identification and merging of his individual Self – Atman – with the Mother, who represents the Spirit – Brahman. This identification of Self and God, Atman and Brahman, which is the teaching of the Advaita Vedantist school, leads to moksha, the freedom or liberation of the Self that is the goal of yoga.

For Vivekananda, highly educated in a Western style, trained as a thinker and rationalist, the path of Jnana Yoga, the yoga of intellectual understanding and penetration into the nature of Reality, was the chosen path. Vivekananda went on to write a very influential book on Raja Yoga, which explained how the beliefs of yoga and science, far from being at odds with each other, could be synthesized. The incidents reported here are from the *Life of Sri Ramakrishna*.

Ramakrishna was born in 1836 of a poor but orthodox Brahmin family. As a child he had an extraordinary memory and could recite long poems and dramas after only a single hearing. He was not scholarly and hated mathematics, but he loved making pottery and painting. He became obsessed with reading about spiritual adepts, and when he read these stories to himself or to others he would fall into a deep meditation. Later, whenever his spiritual feelings were aroused, these meditations would turn into deep trances, and he became open to intense spiritual feelings arising from the beauties of nature.

Although he was a strange child, he had a wonderful spirit that attracted people to him. Neither adults nor children could bear to be separated from him, and his very presence gladdened their heart. At the age of eighteen he was made assistant priest at a temple of the goddess Kali near Calcutta. R. C. Zaehner, in his book *Hinduism*, describes

Ramakrishna's incredible spiritual experiences with the goddess Kali, whom Ramakrishna called 'Mother':

From this moment he fell violently in love with the goddess: there seems no other word for it, though his love was a filial, not a sexual, passion, yet such was its intensity that it left him no peace. He hungered and thirsted after God, his Mother, but his thirst for long remained unsatisfied. He would fall into trances in which all signs of life seemed to have left his body, and so grave did these visitations become that he had to leave the temple. For some twelve years he lived in the woods nearby, tormented by his unsatisfied craving for the divine. At long last he was rewarded by a flash of illumination . . .

Ramakrishna remembered the experience:

I was then suffering from excruciating pain because I had not been blessed with a vision of the Mother. I felt as if my heart were being squeezed like a wet towel. I was overpowered by a great restlessness and a fear that it might not be my lot to realize her in this life. I could not bear the separation any longer; life did not seem worth living. Suddenly my eyes fell on the sword that was kept in the Mother's temple.

Determined to put an end to my life, I jumped up like a madman and seized it, when suddenly the blessed Mother revealed herself to me and I fell unconscious to the floor. What happened after that externally, or how that day or the next passed, I do not know, but within me there was a steady flow of undiluted bliss altogether new, and I felt the presence of the Divine Mother.

In these trance-like states Ramakrishna had powerful religious visions, not only of Hindu gods like the Divine Mother and Krishna, but also of Muhammad and Jesus, both of whom he studied intently. This unusual openness to a wide range of religious experience led him to conclude that all religions must be true, that they were all different paths leading to the same goal – the One, the eternal undivided being which is absolute knowledge and bliss.

His acceptance of all religions and his willingness to teach and embrace all castes and classes, as well as his passionate God-obsessed personality, made Ramakrishna a magnet for a group of young disciples who would take his reformed vision of Hinduism to the outside world, making Hinduism a universal religion to stand alongside the other world religions of Judaism, Christianity, Islam and Buddhism. Since yoga was so essential a part of Hinduism, it too made this world-wide journey.

Ramakrishna had married a little girl of six when he was twenty-five, but she stayed with her parents for thirteen years before joining him, and she then looked after him until his death in 1886. However, Ramakrishna was now a sannyasin, a monk who had taken a vow of chastity, so the marriage was never consummated. Ramakrishna abhorred sexuality, and he saw women, when they were the object of male sexuality, as the arch-enemies of spirituality. He referred to his wife as the 'Holy Mother' and expected his disciples to do the same. I believe this strain of Puritanism can still be felt among some of the schools of yoga today.

Ramakrishna was direct, child-like and emotional, and the strength of his personality, as well as the power of his spiritual experiences, had a striking effect on those who met him. One day, a seventeen-year-old Indian student, Narendra Nath Datta, visited Ramakrishna with some friends.

Narendra Nath was a child prodigy who developed into one of those perfect all-round types that everyone envied in high school: strong in body, agile in mind, a skilled athlete, a good musician, highly sociable and a sharp debater. He combined deep intelligence with a powerful memory and a lively imagination, and was noted for his love of truth, his compassion for the less fortunate, and his independent spirit. Even from childhood, he had a strong religious disposition and taught himself to meditate, which is how he spent much of the night. Coming from a well-placed, educated, middle-class, Westernized family, he was destined for great things, but would they be things of the world or of the spirit?

Every night, as I went to bed, two visions floated before my mind's eye. One of them pictured me as a successful man of the world, occupying the foremost place in society, and I felt that I actually had the power to carve out such a place for myself. A moment later would come the other vision, in which I found myself a wandering monk, dressed in a loincloth, living on chance morsels of food, and spending the night under trees, depending solely on God. I felt that I could lead this sort of life, too.

Narendra was planning on taking a law degree, and was studying history and Western philosophy, whose agnostic doctrines strongly attracted him. A modernist and sceptic, a believer in Western ideas and science, he had no faith in the Hindu gods and laughed at many of the injunctions in the Hindu scriptures. But Narendra was blessed with a strong spiritual foundation, a deep desire to pursue the truth, and he soon found himself in the midst of a spiritual struggle, with his intellect drawn towards the appeal of reason, but his senses wanting a flesh-and-blood reality that could appeal to his soul. It was at this critical moment that he first met Ramakrishna at the holy man's home. Ramakrishna asked him to sing a Bengali song:

I sang the song, but shortly after, he suddenly rose, and taking me by the hand, led me to the northern veranda, shutting the door behind him. It was screened from outside; so we were alone. I thought that he was going to give me some private instructions. But to my utter surprise, he began to shed profuse tears of joy as he held my hand, and addressing me most tenderly as one long familiar to him, said, 'Ah, you come so late! How could you be so unkind as to keep me waiting so long? My ears are well-nigh burnt in listening to the profane talk of worldly people. Oh, I am panting to unburden my mind to one who can appreciate my innermost experiences.'

Thus he went on amid sobs. Then he stood before me with folded palms and began to address me, 'Lord, I know that you are that ancient sage, Nara – the Incarnation of Narayana – born on earth to remove the misery of mankind,' and so on.

I was altogether taken aback by his conduct. 'Who is this that I have come to see?' I thought. 'He must be stark mad! Why, I am but the son of Vishwanath Datta, and yet he dares to address me thus!

I sat and watched him. There was nothing wrong in his words, movements or behaviour towards others. Rather, from his spiritual conversation and ecstatic states he seemed to be a man of genuine renunciation, and there was a marked consistency between his words and life. He said, 'God can be realized. One can see him and talk to him as I am doing with you. But who cares to do so? People shed torrents of tears for their wife and children, for wealth or property, but who does so for the sake of God? If one weeps sincerely for Him, he surely manifests Himself.' As I heard these things, I could not but believe that he was saying them not like an ordinary preacher, but from the depths of his own realization. But I could not reconcile his words with his strange conduct with me. So I concluded that he must be a monomaniac. But I could not help acknowledging the magnitude of his renunciation. 'He may be a madman,' I thought, 'but only the fortunate few can have such renunciation. Even if insane, this man is the holiest of the holy, a true saint, and for that alone he deserves the reverential homage of mankind.'

For a perplexed and uncertain seventeen-year-old student to be told by the forty-six-year old spiritual saint of his day that he was his soul-brother, an incarnation of the sage Nara born on earth to remove the misery of mankind, must have been a mind-boggling revelation. It's no wonder that Narendra thought Ramakrishna a madman. But at the same time, deep down, he must have recognized some truth in what Ramakrishna said. The reason Ramakrishna greeted Narendra with the words, 'You come so late! How could you kept me waiting so long?' is that Ramakrishna had previously seen Narendra as the sage Nara in one of his visions.

A month later Narendra returned for a second visit, and left this account of their meeting.

I found him sitting alone on the small bedstead. He was glad to see me and calling me affectionately to his side, made me sit beside him on the bed. But the next moment I found him overcome with a sort of emotion. Muttering something to himself, with his eyes fixed on me, he slowly drew near me. I thought he might do something queer as on the preceding occasion. But in the twinkling of an eye he placed his right foot on my body. The touch at once gave rise to a novel experience in me. With my eyes open I saw that the walls and everything in the room whirled rapidly and vanished into naught, and the whole universe, together with my individuality, was about to merge in an all-encompassing mysterious void!

I was terribly frightened and thought that I was facing death, for the loss of individuality meant nothing short of that. Unable to control myself, I cried out, 'What is this you are doing to me? I have my parents at home!' He laughed aloud at this and, striking my chest, said, 'All right, let it rest now. Everything will come in time.' The wonder of it was that no sooner had he said this than that strange experience of mine vanished. I was myself again and found everything, within and without the room, as it had been before. All this happened in less time than it takes me to narrate it, but it revolution-ized my mind.

Narendra was amazed at his transformation and loss of rational control at the man's touch, and he wondered if Ramakrishna was a hypnotist, but he knew that his mind was too strong to be influenced in this way. Narendra was in a dilemma about what had happened to him, and tried using his beloved reason to understand the influence this strange mystic had on him, but was unable to fathom it. When he paid a third visit to Ramakrishna he was deter-mined not to be influenced by him again. After strolling in a nearby garden, they sat in the parlour, and the Master fell into a trance. As Narendra watched, Ramakrishna sud-denly touched him and he immediately lost all outward consciousness. When Narendra awoke, he found the Master stroking his chest. Ramakrishna later wrote about what had occurred:

I asked him several questions while he was in that state. I asked him about his antecedents and whereabouts, his mission in this world, and the duration of his mortal life. He dived deep into himself and gave fitting answers to my questions. They only confirmed what I had seen and inferred about him. Those things shall be a secret, but I came to know that he was a sage who had attained perfection, a past master in meditation, and that the day he learned his real nature, he would give up the body by an act of will, through yoga.

Narendra was now convinced that Ramakrishna was not mad, but had a tremendous power working through him, one that commanded the greatest respect. He had never believed that a person needed a guru to realize God, but he now saw that Ramakrishna had the power to aid him in finding his spiritual path. For his part, Ramakrishna was aware of Narendra's pure character and strength of mind, and his potential to become a powerful world figure. He was only concerned that this power be directed spiritually, so that, as the Lord's instrument, Narendra would bring about a spiritual regeneration of mankind. To achieve this, Ramakrishna encouraged Narendra to realize God, his own true Self.

The highly rational and intellectual Vivekananda (as Narendra later became known) had to be shown the way into his Self by Ramakrishna, who broke down the barriers of reason and intellectual pride that were holding Vivekananda back, and showed him how to open himself emotionally to devotion to the Mother, to God. Ramakrishna could sense that Vivekananda's deepest Self wanted an authentic experience of oneness with the highest power, but was unable to achieve it alone.

Ramakrishna had been initiated in the Vedanta order and was a follower of the Advaita Vedanta philosophy, so he naturally encouraged Narendra to read some of the Advaita treatises. The Advaita Vedanta belief is that only one reality exists – Brahman – an impersonal spiritual being from whom everything else emanates. Brahman is absolute, eternal, timeless, unchanging, cannot be seen, heard or felt, has no form or shape and cannot be known in any ordinary way.

However, Brahman has an uncanny and inscrutable power of creation – maya – that makes the entire universe of changing material forms, including all creatures. But all the creations of maya are temporary and unreal, they are in the nature of illusions, because the sole reality is Brahman, One without a second, who is beyond them. Yet all maya's creations are totally infused with the spirit of Brahman, and in human beings this spirit is called Atman, the spiritual essence that we hold deep in our hearts.

The aim of the Advaita Vedantist is to understand that

Atman and Brahman are the same, that they share in the same reality, and by holding exclusively to that reality and dismissing the world as merely a dream, an appearance, to realize the identity of Atman and Brahman, and so to recognize Brahman as the Absolute, the One and only – referred to as That! This identity of the individual spirit – Atman – with the universal spirit – Brahman – means that in our essence we are like this Universal Spirit, and if we call this Higher Spirit God, then we are like God.

Narendra's rational mind and education led him to regard these writings as blasphemous. He thought there was no greater sin in the world than to think of oneself as identical with the Creator. Anyway, he did not trust gurus, because he did not believe that one person needed another to help make that breakthrough to the beyond. In the end, however, he accepted that he needed Ramakrishna to help him, and his final 'surrender' to Ramakrishna, giving up personal control of his will, allowed Ramakrishna to lead him to find his Self, the God within.

One day Ramakrishna tried to convince Narendra of the identity of the individual Self, Atman, with Brahman, but did not succeed. Narendra berated Ramakrishna, saying, 'I am God, you are God, these created things are God – what can be more absurd than this? The sages who wrote such things must be insane.'

Narendra left the room to smoke a cigarette with another disciple and said to him, 'How can that be? This jug is God, this cup is God, whatever we see is God, and we, too, are God! Nothing can be more preposterous!' The two of them laughed at such a stupid idea, and Ramakrishna, in a state of semi-consciousness in his room, came out to join them, carrying his loin cloth under his arm like a child. 'What are you talking about?' he asked, smiling, as he touched Narendra on the arm, plunging himself into samadhi. Narendra described the effect of this touch:

That magic touch of the Master immediately brought a change over my mind. I was stupefied to find that really there was nothing in the universe but God! I saw it quite clearly but kept silent, to see if the idea would last. But that influence did not abate in the course of the day. I returned home, but there too everything I saw appeared to be Brahman. I sat down to take my meal, but found that everything – the food, the plate, the person who served, and even myself – was nothing but That. I ate a morsel or two and sat still. I was startled by my mother's words. 'Why do you sit still? Finish your meal,' and began to eat again. But all the while, whether eating or lying down or going to college, I had the same experience and felt myself always in a sort of comatose state.

While walking in the streets I noticed cabs plying, but I did not feel inclined to move out of the way, for I felt that the cabs and myself were of one stuff. There was no sensation in my limbs which, I thought, were becoming paralysed. I had no satisfaction from eating, and felt as if somebody else was eating. Sometimes I lay down during a meal and after a few minutes got up and began to eat again. The result would be that on some days I would take too much, but it seemed to do no harm. My mother became alarmed and said that there must be something wrong with me. She was afraid that I would not live long.

When this state altered a little, the world began to appear to me as a dream. While walking in Cornwallis Square I would strike my head against the iron railings to see if they were real or only a dream. This state of things continued for some days. When I became normal again, I realized that I must have had a glimpse of the Advaita state. Then it struck me that the word of the scriptures were not false. Thenceforth I could not deny the conclusions of the Advaita philosophy.

Ramakrishna had now fallen mortally ill, and Narendra was involved with others in looking after the holy man as he lay dying. Narendra's desire for the highest truth, the realization of God, now came to him quite unexpectedly.

It was one evening when he was meditating in the house. At first he felt as if a light had been placed behind his head. Then he passed beyond all relativity and was lost in the Absolute. He had attained the Nirvikalpa Samadhi! When he regained a little consciousness of the world, he found only his head, but not his body. He cried out, 'Ah, where is my body?' Hearing this voice, Gopal Senior came into the room. Naren repeated his question. 'Here it is, Naren,' answered Gopal. When that failed to convince Narendra, Gopal was terrified and hastened to inform the Master. The latter only said, 'Let him stay in that state for a while! He has teased me long enough for it!' After a long time, Narendra came to the consciousness of the physical world and found his brother-disciples clustered about him. An ineffable peace bathed his soul.

Vivekenanda's transformation at the hands of Ramakrishna shows us how difficult it is for people brought up and educated in a rational and materialistic philosophy to accept and find the spiritual in themselves. Like Vivekananda, we are taught to be sceptical about all subjective and spiritual experiences, and instead try to effect a wilful control over the world, which damages our minds and bodies. We find it difficult to let go or 'surrender' this control, which we have to do in order to open ourselves to the inner spiritual freedom that is our birthright. The integration or unity of the Self is not something that we can will or deliberately bring about. It is something that must come upon us spontaneously. We need to invite that unity, to entice it to enter us, and it is by practising yoga and learning self-control that we can prepare our body, mind and spirit for this surprising visitation, a blessing that, if we are lucky, can come upon us.

We need to let go of our belief that we can control the world, which is our ultimate illusion. We need to learn the limitations of our will, and when we are able to let go of the will, real thinking and feeling can be released in us and to us. We may not want, or be capable, of handling transcendental experiences like those of Ramakrishna and Vivekananda, but we can understand through such experiences that there is a Beyond that it is important for us to approach.

After being initiated by Ramakrishna into the Vedanta order and being named his spiritual heir, Narendra Nath Datta took the name Swami Vivekananda, and it was through this dedicated, highly intelligent and modern yogi that the practice of yoga was eventually brought to America.

Collecting a small group of disciples around him, Vivekananda organized them into the Ramakrishna Order, and they fanned out throughout India as wandering monks, depending solely on God, in the form of food offerings from others. After five years, Vivekananda realized that trying to teach the people philosophy when they were hungry was no solution, and he reorganized the Order to serve the people, including the untouchables, by providing practical education, medical treatment and food.

Vivekananda accepted Ramakrishna's advice to 'keep the knowledge of Advaita in your pocket, and then act as you like in the world'. He took this advice with him, when in 1893 he was invited to the first World Parliament of Religions in Chicago, and his reception there caused a sensation. This young, dynamic, thoughtful monk presented Hinduism not as a crude and ossifying religion but as a universal faith, as the Mother of Religions, with a message applicable today.

Echoing his Master, Vivekananda spoke of all religions as true. R. C Zaehner summarized his American and European lectures:

. . . he proclaimed from the house-tops the absolute divinity of man . . . Man is by nature free, his liberation is permanently with him, and it is he, no other, who binds himself in illusion: he has within himself the power to cast off his chains, and it is only his attachment to his miserable, unreal ego that prevents him from doing so. 'So when we have nobody to grope towards, no devil to lay our blame upon, no Personal God to carry our burdens, when we are alone responsible, then we shall rise to our highest and best.'

Vivekananda's radical and inspiring message 'put India on the intellectual and religious map of the world, and its huge contribution to thought and religion is now universally admitted'. The interest in Indian culture, and in Vivekananda's own teaching and practices, led to yoga becoming widely disseminated in the West. In spreading this discipline, Vivekananda's influence has come some way towards fulfilling Schopenhauer's prophecy that the spiritual teachings of the yogis 'are destined sooner or later to become the faith of the people'.

Vivekananda and his teacher Ramakrishna have bequeathed to the West a priceless legacy that, if used wisely, can not only transform our personal Selves but also work for the spiritual welfare of our societies. As Jung said, 'The spiritual achievement of the East is one of the greatest things the human mind has ever created.' How we use this golden legacy may well determine the future well-being of our civilization.

12

The Upanishads: *The Secret Teachings*

Unlike the early *Vedas*, such as the *Rig Veda*, the *Upanishads* are not concerned with religious ritual, but with the deeper meaning behind ritual. The anonymous composers of the *Upanishads* maintain an interest in prayer – what is said to the gods – but they are more concerned with profound and searching questions, both physical and metaphysical, such as:

- ◆ What happens to us when we die?
- ◆ Is there one God, or many?
- ◆ If there is one God, what is its nature?
- ◆ Is the universe many things, or is it One?
- ◆ What is the relationship between God and humanity?
- ◆ How did the world come about?
- ◆ What is the world made of?
- ◆ Are we body or spirit?
- ◆ What is the nature of consciousness?
- ◆ What is our purpose in life?

The *Upanishads* are a collection of dialogues, fables, parables and discourses of a spiritual, philosophical and religious nature, and they were composed by a diverse authorship of sages, yogis and rishis, who were some of the earliest seekers of spiritual knowledge. Their investigations were attempts to answer some of the questions listed above and to explain some of the secrets and mysteries of life. Once they gained some understanding, they passed this knowledge on to their students, often in elevated and poetic language. They found a vision of a higher reality and tried to convey their feelings about this reality in a strong emotional language.

The early *Upanishads* were composed sometime between 600 and 400 BCE and they form part of the Vedanta, meaning the end of the *Vedas*. The writings are speculative in that they are a form of imaginative thinking, an attempt to discover some of the profound mysteries of existence. Since these mysteries remain the same now as they were 2,500 years ago, we find ourselves in the same position as students of the *Upanishads*, waiting to hear about these important discoveries. The word *Upanishad* literally means 'at the feet of the Master', which is where we figuratively find ourselves, but its more normal usage is 'secret teachings'.

The teachings are secret in three senses. First, they were esoteric in that they would originally have been oral teachings, passed down from poet to small audience, from seer to seeker, from sage to student. Second, they were secret because they came from deep inside the yogis who composed them, from a place of hidden mystery that borders on the unconscious. Third, they were secret in that, like all true wisdom teachings, the knowledge they express conveys real secrets about the world, true knowledge about how to find wholeness, well-being, contentment – in a word, liberation.

Coming as we do from a tradition of 300 years of scientific rationalism and materialism, it is easy for us to dismiss this internal knowledge as subjective fantasy or imaginative poetry that is ineffective or useless in the external world. It's true that these mystical secrets cannot be verified except by personal experience, but is this any different from the theories of Stephen Hawking and other physicists who imaginatively speculate on the nature of space and the origins of our universe, without any possibility of verifying their ideas? Because they are scientists, we willingly accept the results of their speculations, whereas mystics who speculate on the nature of consciousness and its relation to a higher reality are often looked on as dreamers and fantasists.

Our own contemporary search for meaning demands that we continue to ask the same searching questions as the ancient yogis, because we feel that to answer them, however tentatively, is to place ourselves in some kind of context with the rest of existence, which can take away the isolating and alienating feeling that we are separate, valueless objects placed in an uncaring universe purely by chance. Instead, we need to understand and feel that we are part of a larger web of existence, a unity in which we play an important part, no matter how small, and that this connection gives us a sense of community with other people, nature, and some kind of higher power. In this way, we can free ourselves from existential fear and insecurity and gain a deeper, warmer, more intimate feeling of security, knowing that the world is truly our home, a place that we can share co-operatively and compassionately with others, so that together we are able to extract meaning and purpose from our lives.

To many people, the prospect of finding meaning in a meaningless world feels hopeless or impossible, but the problem of meaning is a universal and perennial one for humanity, and the seers of the *Upanishads* must have been engaged on a similar task, as this parable from the *Katha Upanishad* shows:

> *A person comes to a place where there are two paths ahead: one path is the joy of the essence of one's being, and the other is the path of worldly pleasures. Those that choose the spiritual path connect to their essence, their inner truth, and find*

eventual and perennial peace, while those pursuing immediate pleasures do not.

If you are wise you understand that you have this choice. There is a path of wisdom and a path of ignorance. There are ignorant people who go through life wise only in self-esteem and proud of their learning. They believe that they are their body and that when their body dies, they are gone. But they are deluded.

This choice in life, between the two distinct paths of wisdom and ignorance, faced the Upanishadic writers with the same intensity as it does us today. We need to make a choice, but the path of wisdom seems like a much more difficult path at the beginning. Here is exactly the same choice described as virtue and vice by Xenophon, in a famous parable from Greek times:

Hercules, when he was approaching manhood, went out into the wilderness, and came to a place of two paths. There he sat down, confused as to which of these paths he should choose.

He saw in the distance two giant female figures advancing towards him, one dressed all in white, with an engaging and graceful manner of walking. She was gifted by nature with a slim elegance, a downward look of solemn modesty, and a calm serenity.

The second woman wore a see-through gown and had her face made up to look white and rosy, almost like a mask. She was plump and soft, and her gaze was bold. She glanced from side to side to see if anyone was observing her, and she frequently looked back at her own shadow.

As they approached closer, the elegant woman maintained the same pace, but the second one, bolder and more eager to get to him, ran right up to Hercules and said:

'I see that you are perplexed, Hercules, in choosing which path to take to enter life; if you will be my friend, I can show

you the easiest and most delightful road, on which you can taste every kind of pleasure, and lead a life free from all trouble.

'You shall have no thought of affairs of state, but shall spend your days wondering what kind of rare foods and drink you can find to gratify your appetite, what beautiful objects you can discover to delight your eyes, what harmonious sounds to lull your ears, what sweet odours to smell and what smooth and luxurious objects to stroke. And you will seek many other delightful objects of affection to give you the maximum pleasure that can be found, and at the end of your day you may sleep most softly and dream only pleasant dreams. All of these enjoyments can be found with the least amount of trouble.

'And if you ever feel any anxiety that you will not be able to afford these delights, don't worry that I will force you to procure them by work, or by any suffering of body or mind; but you will be able to enjoy what others have worked for, and you will not restrain yourself from any kind of activity from which it may be possible to find profit, for I give my followers license to seize whatever they want from any source whatsover.'

Hercules said, 'And what, oh beautiful one, is your name?'

'My friends,' she said, 'call me Happiness, but those who dislike me disparage me by giving me the name of Vice.'

Now the second woman had arrived, and she spoke. 'I have also come to speak with you, Hercules, because I have hopes that if you follow the path that leads to my house, you will become an excellent example of whatever is good and meritorious, and through your actions I shall be seen as more valuable and attractive. '

I will not deceive you with promises of pleasure, but must tell you how things really are in this world, and how the gods have set things up. For everything that is valuable and excellent, the gods will not give to mankind without some effort and care; so if you want the gods to be favourable to you, you *must worship them; if you want to be loved by your friends, you must try to serve them and look after their interests; if you desire to be honoured by your city or country, you must benefit them with some advantage; if you feel anxious about the earth yielding you an abundance of fruits for your sustenance, you must cultivate the earth; if you want to enrich yourself with cattle, you must bestow care on those animals; if you are eager to secure freedom for your friends and subdue your enemies, you must learn the arts of war; if you wish to be vigorous in body, you must train your body to obey your mind, and exercise it with effort.'*

Here Vice interrupted and said:

'Do you see, Hercules, how difficult and tedious a road this woman wants you to follow, while I can lead you, by an easy and short path, to perfect happiness?'

The Upanishadic rishis or seers understood that the difficulty in seeking wisdom is that this path requires of the spiritual seeker an act of self-sacrifice, not the external sacrifice of an offering of plants or animals at an altar, but an interior sacrifice of self-denial and self-restraint, a willingness not only to forgo things that are on offer, but to actually give of ourselves, as an offering to life.

Since our society is based on creating desire and a philosophy that encourages people to take without limits rather than give, it seems almost blasphemous to try to reduce desire for material things, and instead to go in search of the spiritual. The act of self-sacrifice means to sacrifice the limited ego or small self, with its narrowness, separation and suffering, and instead discover and realize our true Self, which gives us greater rewards and blessings. This self-sacrifice, which the Hindus call renunciation, is an admission to ourselves that the Spirit is primary, and enables us to discover our true nature or essence, our real Self. Finding this Self takes away fear and gives us courage:

We were given senses to look outward, so many of us only look to the world outside and don't look within ourselves. You can only find your true Self by looking inwards. The ignorant person runs after pleasure and gets caught up in Death's nets. The wise person, understanding that the Eternal Self cannot die, does not chase after worldly pleasures that are impermanent.

When the wise understand that it is only through the Eternal Self that we see, taste, smell, feel, hear and enjoy, they meditate on this Self and go beyond all suffering. When we are present with our Self, we are beyond fear. And this is our true nature.

The Eternal Self lives not only in our hearts but also among the physical elements. It is a boundless power manifesting as life itself, entering every heart, living there among the elements – that is the Eternal Self.

The discovery of the Eternal Self is one of the secrets that the yogis brought back from their internal explorations of consciousness, that universe of vast inner space within us. They brought these secrets back to share with us, to give us an insight into their methods so that we too can duplicate their experiments, if we wish. They were spiritual pioneers on the path to freedom, the first scientific explorers of inner space, and the methods they left for us are still effective, since our deepest inner nature does not change, no matter how much societies, technologies and all external factors do. The nature of our nature is the first secret lesson they left for us, and the Upanishads represent a treasury of wisdom that can help us find a way out of perplexity and alienation and into meaning. They uttered a truth that is everlasting, and this truth is the vital secret of how to find freedom and peace.

If the ancient sages saw themselves as scientists and explorers, the first object that they investigated was the mind itself, and the nature of consciousness. Here is what the yogi who composed the *Mandukya Upanishad* discovered over 2,000 years ago about states of consciousness:

> *There is nothing that is not Spirit. Your inner Self is also Spirit, self-same, identical, and it exists in four states:*
>
> *The first is the waking life, called Vaishvamnara, when our consciousness turns outward through the senses, focused only on the material world.*
>
> *The second is the dreaming state, Taijasa, the shining one, when our senses are turned inward, and we re-enact the subtle and luminous impressions of past deeds, present desires and fears of the future.*
>
> *The third is deep sleep, Prajna, the all-knowing, when there are neither dreams nor desires. The mind switches off in Prajna, and there is no experience of separateness, but the sleeper is unaware of this. If the sleeper can become conscious while still in deep sleep, then the door to peace and joy opens.*
>
> *The fourth condition is super-consciousness, called Turiya, pure awareness, when a person is neither inward nor outward, and is beyond the senses and the intellect: he is in fact nothing more than the individual Real Self, called Atman. He realizes the supreme goal of life: infinite peace and love. Realize your true Self, the peaceful, blissful Atman.*

The yogi in a state of deep meditation observed his consciousness and found four different states or conditions: waking, dreaming, dreamless sleep and the fourth – a super-conscious state called turiya – which later yogis called samadhi and the Buddha called nirvana. When, over 2,000 years after this discovery, technologists created a machine capable of taking readings of brain activity through attaching electrodes to the head, scientists reported that they found four different wave patterns, which they called alpha, beta, theta and delta. These four wave patterns coincide exactly with the yogi's own 'brain scan' and show that his scientific method was quite adequate for the task in hand. The fourth state – Turiya – equates with the alpha state of deep relaxation.

The yogi understood very well what the waking, dreaming and dreamless states were, because they are common to us all. But unlike the machine, which can only give print-outs of data, this ancient human brain scanner was able to make observations and gain insights that led to a new discovery:

If the sleeper can become conscious while still in deep sleep, then the door to peace and joy opens.

Have you ever woken up, actually become conscious, while still in deep sleep? I have, and it's an amazing feeling. Sometimes, in the middle of the afternoon, I take a short nap if I feel my concentration waning. I lie down on a couch, and after five or so minutes manage to fall asleep, and once or twice during such naps I have found myself becoming aware that I am conscious, even though I am still asleep. I know that I am sleeping, because my body feels beyond my control – I have only vague sensations of things outside me, I can't move my limbs, and I can't even open my eyes. So I stay in this state of sleep/awareness, watching and observing, since there is nothing I can 'do'.

The image that I have of this experience is not easy to describe, but it feels as if my awareness, which is still a vague sense of 'I', is spread out over an area rather than focused on a subject. My awareness does not feel at all directed since there is nothing to 'see', but is just somehow there, existing, observing, a kind of background consciousness. This diffuse awareness feels like the inner membrane of an egg, or even the inner lining of the nucleus of a cell, and it seems to have a vague sense of the curvature of such a membrane. There is really no object for this awareness to focus on, there is no egg or nucleus to observe, but in the virtual space where the 'egg' would be, there is only the feeling of awareness of itself. I can only assume that this awareness of an observing but non-doing 'I' is an experience of my 'Self'.

This state of pure awareness or super-consciousness is the fourth state – turiya – that the yogi discovered, and since it leads to such a pleasant feeling, he wants to discover a method to find it again, not just by relying on accidental means. But why should he want to enter this state?

Beyond the senses are the objects of desire, beyond the objects of desire is the mind, beyond the mind is the intellect, beyond the intellect is our true nature and our true Self. Beyond the true Self is the Eternal Spirit of the universe. This is where the path ends.

The light of the Eternal Spirit is invisible and hidden in everyone. It is seen only by those who keep their mind concentrated on love and thus develop a super-conscious manner of knowing. Meditation enables them to go deeper and deeper into consciousness, from the world of words to the world of thoughts and then beyond thoughts to the wisdom in the Self, able to find inner peace.

This Eternal Self is formless and can never be seen with the eyes. But it is revealed in your heart when it is purified through meditation and the stilling of the senses. When the five senses and the mind are still, and the ego itself rests in silence, then your spiritual journey begins. This calm steadiness of the senses is called yoga, the union of mind, body and spirit. When one can stay in the state of union, the yogi can do no wrong. Before this state is reached, the unity of yoga comes and goes.

Through meditation, the yogi achieves a state of unity, or integration, a state of inner peace called yoga, and through this deep yogic meditation he finds a way to still his senses and his active mind, and in this silence he is rewarded with a new vision, a new revelation – his inner essence, the silent watcher which he calls his Self. And beyond this Self he 'sees' the light of the Spirit, something great that is beyond his individuality. He accomplishes these new discoveries though a technique or method of concentration that the composer of the *Shvetashvatara Upanishad* describes:

> *Sit with your spine erect and lead your mind and your senses inward; use the mantra OM and let it echo in your heart, freeing you from fear and sorrow. When your body becomes silent and steady, breathing rhythmically through the nose, you can train your senses to be quiet. The chariot of the mind is drawn by wild horses and those wild horses have to be tamed.*
>
> *Choose a clean, quiet and cool place for meditation and the practice of yoga, where the sound of dancing water and the beauty of the place foster thought and contemplation. In deep meditation you may see forms like snow or smoke, you may feel a strong wind blowing or a wave of heat, or you may see more and more light within. These are signs that you are on the spiritual path to reach the Eternal Spirit of Brahman.*

The yogis made the discovery that our essence is not body and mind, but is really Spirit, and they set out to discover the nature of this Spirit. In the *Upanishads* they mainly use two terms to refer to the spirit: Atman and Brahman, which we translate as Self and Spirit respectively. Brahman – Spirit – is the impersonal principle or source of everything, and is considered absolute, eternal, infinite, indivisible. It is the One in All and the All in One, and so on. Brahman is the same as the Tao of the Taoists, the Great Spirit of the American Indians, and the Godhead beyond God in the Judeo-Christian tradition. It is the highest power conceivable, beyond all opposites, beyond time and space, and is the source of all creation,

It is fire, sun, moon and stars. It is the air and the sea; it is this boy, that girl, this man, that woman, this old man – its face is everywhere. It is the blue bird, the green bird, the thundercloud, the seasons and the seas. It has no beginning and no end. It is the Creator, the source from which the worlds evolve, and Its face is everywhere. The magic of name and form, of you and me, casting the spell of pain and pleasure, all come from maya, its Divine power. It is only when we are able to see through this magic veil that we can see the One who appears as many.

Our visible and phenomenal world, the world of Nature, is the creation of Brahman produced through maya, his 'uncanny power', but Brahman is not a transcendent God like the Hebrew God YHWH, who stands outside of nature and creates the universe like a potter moulding clay. For the yogis, the world we inhabit is made from Brahman itself, it is an emanation of its Being, so that Brahman is both transcendental, meaning beyond, and imminent, meaning infused. Brahman is both creator and created, both outside and inside. The yogi tries to see behind the material appearance of things, including his own body and mind, to reveal the spiritual Reality of Brahman. The *Brihadaranyaka* and *Shvetashvatara Upanishads* tell it like this:

A wife loves her husband, but it is not for the love of her husband that her husband is dear, but for the Spirit that is in the husband. It is the same for children, wives, wealth, religion, power, animals, and everything else. Nothing is loved for its own sake, it is only the Self, or Spirit that is loved. When this Self or Spirit is seen and heard in our thoughts and meditation, then we know and understand everything that exists.

When you look into another person's eyes what you see is the Self, fearless and deathless. That is the Higher Spirit, Brahman, the Supreme.

Brahman, the Supreme Spirit, infuses everything that is created with Spirit, so that everything in the universe is Brahman. In human beings, the rishis call that same Spirit Atman, the Eternal Self, but the Upanishadic writers make the point that Atman and Brahman, Self and Spirit, must be the same, identical in every way, equally infinite and eternal, since Spirit is indivisible. Juan Mascaro in his introduction to the *Upanishads* says of this:

Thus the momentous statement is made in the Upanishads that God must not be sought as something far away, separate from us, but rather as the very inmost of us, as the higher Self in us above the limitations of our little self. In rising to the best in us we rise to the Self in us, to Brahman, to God himself.

The sages believed that beyond the material world, and this is the reason why the material world exists at all, there is something that represents real existence. And this something they discovered to be not far away in space, but within us, inside our inner space, where it can be easily discovered. This idea of a Spirit or divinity within gives us the possibility of becoming God-like, of finding that we are capable of aspiring to and expressing universal qualities of truth and love, qualities that we might otherwise reserve for the gods. The *Chandogya Upanishad* says:

In the centre of the castle of the Infinite Spirit, which is Brahman, in our own body, there is a small shrine shaped like a lotus flower in which there is a small space. We need to find out who lives there and we should desire to know Him. Why is it so important?

Because this little space within our hearts is as great as the whole vast world outside. Heaven, earth, fire, wind, the sun, moon and stars; whatever is and whatever is not, everything

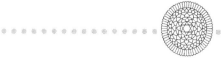

is there, for the whole universe is in Him and He dwells in our hearts.

The Spirit that lives in that space does not grow old and die. No one can ever kill the Spirit that is everlasting. The love of the universe dwells in the real castle of the Spirit, which we call Brahman. The Self, the Atman, desires only what is real, and thinks nothing but what is true.

Atman, the Self, is pure, free from decay and death, free from hunger and thirst and free from sorrow. This is the Spirit in man. The only thing this Spirit desires is truth. This is the Spirit that we must seek and know: we must each find our own Self. When we have found our Self and got to know it, we have reached the ultimate, and there is nothing more to desire.

The aim of the Upanishadic yogis and the later followers of Vedanta philosophy, which was based on the *Upanishads*, was to realize the Self, and to them this meant not just understanding intellectually that Self and Spirit, Atman and Brahman, are the same, but actually experiencing and embodying that identification in themselves through yoga and meditation. External knowledge and learning were not enough, they required that a sympathetic union of Self and Spirit take place. This identification of Self and Spirit is the same experience that we saw Sri Ramakrishna and Swami Vivekananda recount some 2,300 years after it was first reported in the *Chandogya Upanishad*:

It is true that the body will die, but within the body lives the imperishable Self. The body experiences pleasure and pain, so no one that is ruled by his body can ever be free from pleasure and pain. But those that know they are not the body can pass beyond pleasure and pain to live in a state of joy.

The wind, clouds, thunder and lightning have no body, but when they rise up and reach the light, they show their own shapes. Likewise, when the Self is in silent quietness it arises, leaves the body and, reaching the Spirit supreme, finds its body of light. This is the land of infinite liberty where, beyond the mortal body, the Spirit of man is free. There he can laugh and sing and forget that while he was on earth, he was attached to his body. As a beast is attached to a cart, so on earth the Self is attached to a body.

Braman and Atman, Spirit and Self, are represented by the sacred syllable OM, which is chanted at the beginning and end of prayers. The sound of OM is the sound of the Eternal Spirit as well as the essence of speech, and to chant OM is to realize the highest Spirit in one's body and mind:

The word OM is both the transcendent and the immanent highest spiritual power. By chanting this sacred word, the wise connect to this highest power.

OM has three sounds – A, U, M. Those that meditate on the first sound – A – will be born again on this earth to lead a pure life, full of love and faith. Those who meditate on the first two sounds – A and U – go to the lunar world, and after enjoying their heavenly joys, come back to earth again. But if, by meditating on the three sounds of the eternal OM – A, U, M – the wise person puts his mind in meditation upon the Supreme Spirit, he enters the regions of the full light of the sun, where he is freed from all evil and is connected to the highest Spirit.

If the three sounds are not used together, you are led again to life that dies. When the whole mantra – A, U and M – are used together, indivisible and interdependent, the sound reverberates in the mind and, whether awake or asleep, one is freed from fear, and enters into infinite peace.

Om

OM in fact has four sounds, the three main ones – A, U, M – and a lingering and resonating fourth as M turns into N, which fades away slowly into silence, into the ineffable. Many people who practise yoga find the chanting of OM and other Sanskrit words or sayings a bit too exotic or alien to their taste. Not only does chanting feel strange at first, but chanting words from a different religious tradition can feel uncomfortable. It's worth reflecting on the fact that OM has a very close relationship with Amen, as the musician Hazrat Inayat Khan explains in his book, *The Music of Life*:

The words om, omen, amen and amin, which are spoken in all houses of prayer, are of the same origin.

Amen, like OM, is a sacred utterance, and it is a symbol of the Supreme Reality, the highest power that we can conceive of, the power of creation itself. When we chant OM, the sound resonates throughout our bodies, vibrating down into our cells, and helps to shake up the accumulated blockages and toxins that clog up our body. Chanting OM is good for your health, which is one reason why the yogis practise it, and it forms the basis of Mantra Yoga, the repetition of sacred sounds, as Khan explains:

It is the power of the word that works upon each atom of the body, making it sonorous, making it a medium of communication between the external life and the inner life.

Chanting OM is a breathing exercise that sends powerful vibrations through the deepest parts of the body, parts that asanas and ordinary pranayama do not usually reach. These vibrations, besides helping to cleanse our organs and cells, are said to wake up the kundalini, the coiled, creative, serpent power that sleeps at the base of the spine. This primal animal energy is asleep in most of us, because our early conditioning and the life we lead have put it to sleep. But the yogis believe that it can be roused, and once it awakes, it makes a journey up the sushumna, which is the energy channel running within our spine.

Khan talks about why the yogis see this energy as a serpent:

The yogis have learned very much about the secret of breath from the serpent; that is why they regard the serpent as the symbol of wisdom. Shiva, the lord of yogis, has a serpent around his neck as a necklace. It is the sign of mystery, of wisdom. There are cobras in the forests of tropical countries which sleep for six weeks. Then one day the cobra wakens, and it breathes because it is hungry; it wants to eat. Its thoughts attract food from wherever it may be; food is attracted from miles away by its thoughts.

The serpent, too, is so strongly built that without wings it flies and without feet it walks. Also, if there is any animal that can be called the healthiest animal of all, it is the serpent. It is never ill; before it becomes ill, it dies, yet it lives a long time.

The mystics have studied the life of the cobra and they have found two wonderful things. One is that it does not waste energy. Birds fly until they are tired; animals run here and there. The cobra does not do so. It makes a hole where it lives and rests. It knows the best way of repose, a repose that it can continue as long as it wishes.

The natural breathing capacity of the cobra is such as no

other creature shows. That capacity goes as a straight line throughout its body. The current that it gets from space and that runs through it gives it lightness and energy and radiance and power. Compared with the cobra, all other creatures are awkwardly built. The skin of the cobra is so very soft and of such silky texture, and in a moment's time it can shed its skin and be new, just as if born anew.

No doubt the yogis made the connection between the shape of our spine and the shape of the snake, so they visualized the kundalini energy snaking itself up the sushumna; as it does so, it wakes up each of the six energy centres located in the subtle body. These dynamic energy centres are called the chakras, chakra meaning wheel in Sanskrit, and they each relate to a different body system, set of glands and emotional state. The chakras are, from the bottom of the torso to the top of the head: Muladhara, the base chakra, related to excretion; Svadhisthana, the sacral chakra, related to reproduction; Manipura, the solar plexus chakra, related to digestion; Anahata, the heart chakra, related to circulation; Visuddha, the throat chakra, related to respiration, and Ajna, the brow chakra, related to cognition. Above these six is the 1,000-petalled lotus at the crown of the head – the Sahasrara chakra, relating to the brain.

Once the yogi wakes the serpent, actualizes its tremendous electrical power and realizes his Self, he has found the real and the true, and gained inner freedom. His explorations of inner space have brought him to a liberated state that brings with it a feeling of bliss or joy, ending all his suffering and fear,

When the yogi has full power over his body, he can increase the spiritual fire within, giving better health, a light body and freedom from craving. When a gold mirror is covered with dust, it shines again when it has been cleaned. When you have

been cleansed with the truth of the Spirit your life is fulfilled and you are beyond suffering. Then you become a lamp by which you find the truth of the Spirit and see the pure Everlasting Spirit, freeing you from all bondage.

This is the Spirit whose light illumines all creation, the creator of all from the beginning. He was, he is and always shall be; he is in all and sees all. Let us adore the Lord of life who is ever present in fire, water, plants and trees.

The yogis who composed the *Upanishads* were among the first explorers of inner space and they mapped out for us the unknown territory they discovered, conveyed to us a method for continuing and repeating their experiments and brought back for us the most amazing knowledge: that the meaning and wholeness we seek (which some call God) is not to be found in the heavens, or in scriptures, or in ritual, or in some distant land, but is right here within us, just waiting to be discovered. However, they left us with the main responsibility – that of making the decision to follow them. The two paths that they found – ignorance and wisdom – face us every day of our lives. The decision we make as to which path we choose determines our character and our destiny.

When Jews celebrate together, the toast they make is 'L'Chaim' – 'To Life' – and this decision always to choose life means to choose the path of spiritual life rather than death, to choose light rather than darkness, always to try to do the right thing, and in all of life to seek out and follow the truth of our own being, as far as we are able. This saying comes from Deuteronomy:

Life and death I place before you, blessing and curse. Now choose life, so that you may stay alive, you and your descendents.

It is only by following the path of truth and life that we can find any happiness, satisfaction and meaning in life.

13

The Search for Wholeness

S wami Nikhilananda, in his book *Self-Knowledge*, has written:

Self-knowledge is vital. All other forms of knowledge are of secondary importance; for a man's actions, feeling, reasoning, and thinking are dependent upon his idea of the Self.

His view of life will be either materialistic or spiritual according to his conception of himself. If he regards himself as a physical creature, and his soul (provided he believes in such a thing) as subservient to material ends, then he is a materialist; he follows the ideal of material happiness, devoting himself to the attainment of power and the enjoyment of material pleasures. Whenever a large number of people follow such an ideal, society becomes materialistic and there ensue bloodshed, war and destruction.

If, on the other hand, a man regards himself as a spiritual entity and believes that his material body should be utilized to serve a spiritual end, then he is spiritual. He follows the path of unselfishness, consecration and love, and thus becomes a force to promote peace and happiness for all.

Carl Jung saw modern life as progress and liberation, but in the process of change we have allowed our culture to be set adrift from its spiritual roots. Our exclusive cultivation of scientific rationality and technology has led to a one-sided development that focuses our attention on the external world at the expense of the inner life of the Spirit. The result of this narrow concentration is, in his words, a 'breathless drive for power and aggrandisement', ignoring the more important inner values that nourish caring relationships and life itself. No one in our society now has time for self-knowledge or believes that it would serve any good purpose. We have a strong belief in doing, but not in asking about the state of mind and soul of the doer.

Many people now are searching for an inner truth that can sustain them, one they can live by, but this kind of truth is not easy to find or maintain in a society that positively discourages its discovery. Our dominant culture is anti-spiritual because of the threat that true spirituality, passionate emotions and spontaneity pose to its continuation. Our institutions and social practices demean or repress our thirst for true meaning, and this repression leads to harmful stresses and illnesses in daily life, as well as an attitude towards nature that threatens us with ecological disaster.

Sitting isolated as voyeurs in our homes, bombarded by images that convey an ideology of individualism, we see ourselves as alone and separate, islands of isolated consciousness and feeling trying to survive in a hostile world. We see ourselves in competition with others for the things that we think (and have been told) will give us security and happiness. So we buy things and accumulate money that we hope will make us impregnable and give us protection in our fortress of the ego. But our accumulation doesn't end up giving us security; paradoxically it increases fear, because we are now surrounded by possessions that we don't want to lose. Isolated, insecure and afraid, we act increasingly out of our alienation. That alienation creates a permanent stress that builds up tensions in mind, nerves and muscles, pervading down to our cells. This inner tension leads to increased rigidity, a rigidity that is opposed to life and is associated with illness and death.

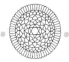

Peter Gabel, in his book *The Bank Teller and Other Essays on the Politics of Meaning*, writes of our desire to escape from this rigidity, fear and isolation:

Every morning, every one of us wakes up with the desire to overcome our isolation and connect with others in a meaningful, life-giving, passionate way. We long for the sense of confirmation and validation that can only come from participation in real community. As we peer out at the day in front of us, however, we feel compelled to suppress this desire, to actually forget about it as best we can, because we have become resigned to the fact that no one else seems to want what each of us wants.

Having grown accustomed to a life deadened by bureaucratic work and family routines, to passing people on the street whose blank gazes seem to indicate an inner absence, we each internalize the sense that in order to feel part of what little community there is in the world we must deny our deepest needs and adjust to things as they are. And so we don our various social masks and become 'one of the others', in part by keeping others at the same distance we believe they are keeping us. In this way, social reality takes the form of a 'circle of collective denial' through which each of us becomes both agent and victim of an infinitely rotating system of social alienation. Trapped in this alienation, people in the West are often unable to imagine themselves acting to change things, no matter how deeply they may desire a different kind of world.

We would like to live in a different way, but four things stop us from attempting to change ourselves, and therefore our world. First, we see other people acting only in their own self-interest, and so assume that they, like everyone else in society, subscribe to the state religion of consumerism and competition. This leads us to believe, wrongly, that we are only one of a small minority who desire change. We do not trust our inner voice, our Self, that encourages us to seek community with others, because our Self knows intuitively that if we feel this way, others must be feeling the same and a similar inhibition holds back their going public with these feelings.

Second, the desire not to be hurt encourages us to keep our desire for meaningful connection to ourselves. We are afraid to reach out to others because we fear the humiliation of rejection, and so we live with a divided Self, both desiring a real link with others and afraid of making the first move to achieve it.

Third, we are pessimistic about change, and believe that our individual efforts are too puny to have any real effect. Consequently, instead of making whatever contribution we can, no matter how small, and feeling good that we have made an effort, we sink back into apathy and allow everything to slide. We fail to understand that the world is not static but is constantly undergoing change, and that a multitude of small changes eventually constitute a greater one.

Fourth, we fear the very change we desire, since our ego has accommodated its security to a set of habitual reactions and does not want to let go of these. Our longing for security at any cost brings on fear when we attempt to break out of our habitual routines. The ego wants to keep tight control, even when we know, deep down, that control is not ours to keep and is even causing the problem. We need to trust the universe, to let go into a process of change, to accept the new and enjoy it, since in doing so we discover our long-lost freedom.

Gabel writes:

By recovering one's authentic being by recognizing yourself as fully human, it is possible to break through the alienation that society places us in. The underlying fear of domination and humiliation by the other is overcome, and a real connection with oneself and other people becomes possible.

To 'recover one's authentic being', to find wholeness and integrity, to transform oneself into a full and vibrant personality, to make a real connection to others, is something that yoga can do for us, and it has been successfully doing this for thousands of years, as the classic text the *Bhagavad Gita* shows.

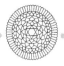

14

A Conversation with God

It is tempting to consider our psychic conflicts and mental suffering as exclusively modern ailments, but the *Bhagavad Gita*, the *Celestial Song*, composed around 500 BCE, shows us that the divided self was a phenomenon known in ancient times. This eighteen-chapter poem, a short interlude in the immensely long Hindu epic, the *Mahabharata*, is a handbook or guide to resolve internal conflicts and to find Self-realization. The *Gita* is the best-loved of all Hindu scriptures, and has been translated into English and other languages hundreds of times. It was Gandhi's favourite, and his inspiration.

The *Gita* consists of a long dialogue between two men: the warrior Prince Arjuna and the God Krishna, and it takes place on a battlefield just before a deadly fight between two sides of the same warring family. The conversation revolves around the conflict in Arjuna, a member of the warrior caste who leads one of the armies, and who is torn about the prospect of killing his relatives and close friends. Arjuna is in a state of spiritual war and peace, one of inner turmoil, and has no idea how to proceed.

As the poem begins, the war is just about to begin, and Arjuna asks Krishna, who is acting as his chariot driver, to wheel him to the centre of the battlefield to look at his enemies, who are also his kinsmen. Arjuna sinks down in despair, throws away his bow and arrows and declares his unwillingness to fight. Whichever way Arjuna chooses, he loses: to fight is to kill those he loves and admires, while refusing to fight, for a warrior, is shameful. It is at this point that Krishna offers him advice. Krishna is an *avatar*, or personalization, of God, who has come down to earth to offer his help in a time of crisis, a bit like Superman,

> *I am the Spirit that dwells in the heart of all things. I am the beginning, the middle and the end of all that lives.*
>
> *I appear to take birth through maya, my own power of illusion. When righteousness is lost and evil prevails, I manifest on earth in bodily form; I come into being from age to age to protect the good, destroy the wicked and establish righteousness.*

The idea of God being available to help humanity in times of crisis is echoed in the Hebrew Bible, when YHWH assures Moses, 'When you need me, I will be there.' And the belief in Jesus as an emissary from God fulfils the same idea.

Krishna now marshals all the arguments why Arjuna must fight, no matter how much it hurts him to do so. Arjuna's conflict is not presented as a realistic war story, concerned with the moral dilemma of if and when violence is necessary, but as an allegory of the soul, a fight between Arjuna's internal forces of darkness and light, the human and the divine, the higher and lower desires, and how to resolve this conflict through yoga.

As we have seen, there are two forces in human life, one pulling us upwards towards spiritual growth, and one dragging us down with the weight of past conditioning. Each one of us has the ability to choose a path in life to pursue: the selfish path leading to confusion and pain, or the unselfish path leading to wisdom and well-being. It is this choice that always faces us, in every generation. How we respond to life's events, how we decide which path to pursue, determines not only our individual destiny, but that of society as a whole.

What is most surprising about the *Gita* is that we are

presented with God, in the form of Krishna, actually offering us advice about how to live. Although the advice here begins as specific counsel for Arjuna in his dilemma, it soon becomes obvious that Krishna is talking about universal values, and about life in a general sense. Krishna's advice is meant for us as well as for Arjuna; whether we listen to it and take up his suggestions is a whole other matter, but it is not often that we are addressed directly by God.

Since Krishna is Spirit taking on a material body, he is unable to act for Arjuna, or for us. Instead, all-knowing, he gives us advice about how best to act in the world, with the aim of resolving our conflicts and restoring health to our divided Self.

Because so many diverse personalities exist in the world, there is no 'one size fits all' yoga, but a variety of approaches are used to cover people's differing souls. Krishna describes a triple yogic path of action, knowledge and devotion that Arjuna can follow in his search for resolution of his mental turmoil. These paths are represented by three spiritual methods: Karma Yoga, Jnana Yoga and Bhakti Yoga. These are all different facets of yoga, Karma Yoga relating to self-less action in the world, Jnana Yoga to a search for wisdom, and Bhakti Yoga expressing love and devotion to God.

Each of these practices appeals to different types of people, and although they are presented as separate and individual yogas, it is clear that there is a merging and inter-penetration between them, and none of them is a stand-alone practice, divorced from the others. Their ultimate aim is also the same – moksha, or freedom of the Self.

The first practice that Krishna offers to Arjuna is Karma Yoga, the yoga of action in the world:

Do your work but don't go looking for any benefits from the results. Don't be motivated by the fruits of your actions, but you must never become inactive either.

This teaching is quite radical, because it tells us not to act in the world for ourselves, but selflessly, for others. We must act, says Krishna, we have no choice, but if we act according to selfish desires, through attachment, we will not find peace.

Do your work in the peace of yoga, free from selfish desires, not being moved by success or failure. Yoga is evenness of the mind, a peace that is always steady. Work done for reward is much lower than work done through the yoga of wisdom.

Karma Yoga is action in the world, something that we all understand, because our survival forces us to act. But the fear of poverty, and the pressures we feel to conform to a model of success, lead almost all of us to act contrary to Krishna's advice. We do act selfishly, we do worry about outcomes, we do expect rewards, and deep down we suspect that Krishna is probably right, but we lack the courage to try to live up to this ideal. In the *Gita*, an all-knowing God tells us that this is the way to act, that it will not lead to pain and suffering but to joy, but we lack the trust and faith to attempt it, and so ignore this advice.

We live by the Law of Matter, which says that to give away something is to reduce what we have. If I give away some of my money, I have less than before, so I feel poorer. Unfortunately, because we have lost much of our spiritual intelligence, we now apply this law indiscriminately to include spiritual things as well, even though the Law of Matter does not apply in this realm. In the spiritual world there is a different approach, the Law of Spirit, which says that to give away is not to lose, but even to increase what we have. If I offer compassion, tenderness or love, or help someone in need, my store of these is not reduced or diminished, but is returned to me with a bonus. As the *Isha Upanishad* says,

All this is full
All that is full
From fullness, fullness comes
When fullness is taken from fullness
Fullness still remains.

The Law of Spirit says that to give is to increase, and what Krishna is saying to Arjuna is that everything only appears to be material, but all things are in their essence spiritual, and if we treat material things by the Law of Matter, we misunderstand their true nature, and so make mistakes in life. We are once more in the land of avidya – ignorance, or misconception. As someone once wrote,

We are spiritual beings having a human experience, not human beings having a spiritual experience.

What is more material than a building made of bricks, wood and nails – the dense, hard and gritty stuff of the world? But a building was once a blueprint, made of fairly insubstantial paper, and before that it was a concept or idea in the mind of an architect. Now, ideas are spiritual in nature, so a building is really a frozen idea, a bit of spirit made solid by work – human action.

Can we understand that this applies equally to all other objects, including money, which is just a material symbol created by us to mark a transaction, a temporary relationship between people? Krishna wants us to see that our possessions and money are just material forms of spirit, and that the Law of Spirit, rather than the Law of Matter, applies to them.

The ability to see things in their true nature, not clouded over by convention, selfish desires or ego, is a training of Jnana Yoga, which is the second practice Krishna offers. This second step continues the path of action, Karma Yoga, but broadens and deepens it to become one with the path of knowledge – Jnana Yoga. This is the path to Self-realization and the inner knowledge of the true nature of the Self and the world.

This yogic practice trains us, in meditation, to look deeply into things, to penetrate their essence, so that we are able to understand what really happens in action. This uncovers another of the reasons why we should act without expectation of rewards or benefits, because we see that the results of our actions have not been caused by us. The Chinese have a saying that reflects this situation:

Care only for ploughing and weeding, ask not for the harvest.

We act by planting the seed and weeding around it, but the growth and development of the plant are not our doing. It is Nature, not our action, that provides the harvest, and we need to know where our will ends and the force of Nature takes over.

The force of Nature does everything that is accomplished. But when our minds are clouded with ego, we think that we have made things happen.

Through acting without selfish desires, and understanding that the results of our actions are not down to us, but are really the effects of Nature's work, we realize that our true Self, though inactive, is the equal of these powerful forces of Nature. By taking away the false pride of personal accomplishment, which can lead to arrogance, we gain a feeling of true inner Self-confidence, leading to a state of steady wisdom.

The sages say that whoever does things without personal desire for success is wise. That person's actions are pure and he knows the truth. In whatever work he does, such a man has peace: he expects nothing, and he relies on nothing. He does nothing, although he is always engaged in action. Having given up desire, with control over his mind and ego, he is free from all attachments, and only his body works. He is free from sin. He is happy with whatever the universe has given him and is not attached to pleasure or pain; he is happy whether he succeeds or not, and is not bound by his actions. When you let go of all attachments and experience liberation, you find peace in wisdom.

A person who has been able to let go of all personal desires and is completely content in the truth of his Self, is someone whose soul has found peace. A person whose mind is not troubled by sorrows and has no longing for pleasure and happiness, who is beyond passion, fear and anger – that is someone of steady wisdom. One who is free of all mental attachments and neither rejoices when good things happen, nor feels repelled when bad happens, maintains a serene wisdom.

Krishna advises us that the way to stay selflessly centred in Karma Yoga, and to find the steady wisdom of Jnana Yoga, is to learn to withdraw from the objects of sense, the same teaching that the *Yoga Sutras* calls pratyahara, the fifth limb of the ashtanga system, as described by Patanjali:

When our mind is withdrawn from sense objects, the sense organs also withdraw themselves from their respective objects and are said to imitate the mind. This is known as pratyahara. Then we have complete mastery over our senses.

Krishna describes it as follows:

The person who can withdraw his senses from the attractions of the pleasures of sense, like a tortoise drawing its limbs within its shell, his wisdom is unwavering. When we stop

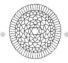

feeding on sense objects, they drop away, but the longing for them doesn't. But even that longing disappears when our Self connects with its highest truth. Even for the wise, if their senses become excited, their minds get carried away too.

It is through the third practice, that of Bhakti Yoga, the yoga of devotion or love of God, that Arjuna is taught to control his senses, just as the *Yoga Sutras* explained that controlling the mind is the goal of yoga practice. Krishna says:

The yogi learns to control the senses by meditating on me as the highest goal. Because his senses are controlled, his wisdom again becomes steady. When a person dwells on the pleasures of the senses, he develops an attachment to them; this attachment leads to desire and desire results in anger. Anger gives rise to confusion and confusion to loss of memory. When we lose our memory, we lose our powers of reasoning, and when reason is gone, we are absolutely lost.

But the yogi who has disciplined the mind and has gained control of his senses is free from attraction and aversion, and can settle deeply in serenity. In that serenity, his sorrows disappear; for then the heart has found tranquillity, wisdom and peace.

You cannot find wisdom or meditate if the senses are out of control. Without this contemplation there cannot be peace, and without peace there is no joy. The mind that follows the wandering senses loses all reason, like a ship that is tossed about on rough seas.

We cannot experience true peace when we have desires. But when all desires merge like rivers flowing into the ocean, we are ever one in infinite peace.

Anyone can experience peace if you live without personal desires, free of 'mineness' and egoism.

Jnana Yoga gave us the wisdom to understand that the results of our actions are not really ours, but are benefits created by the force of Nature. By meditating further in Jnana Yoga we are able to trace Nature back to its source and discover that the Spirit, Krishna, is the true power behind that force. And since Krishna, the highest power, is also the source of our life and whatever power we have, we understand the oneness that connects our actions to nature and to the Spirit.

So in this third step, all three are united: the Karma Yoga of actions continues, the knowledge and wisdom of Jnana Yoga expands, and we add Bhakti Yoga, devotion, to the mix. Bhakti Yoga involves the adoration of our true Self as the Highest Spirit. Our inner Self is seen to be the same as the Spirit that governs Nature, and that directs all of our actions, perfectly transcendent, through Nature. We recognize the Spirit, Krishna, as the source and power behind all things:

I am the Spirit that dwells in the heart of all things. I am the beginning, the middle and the end of all that lives. Among creators, I am the creator of Love; I am the knowledge of the Self that makes ignorance disappear. I am the splendour in all that is splendid. I am the goodness of those who are good. There is no end to my manifestations. Know that all things beautiful and good, prospering or powerful, are only a small portion of my radiance.

The Highest Spirit is the source of everything, including our own Self, and is the origin of everything we hold dear: life, love and goodness. To this Highest Spirit, Krishna asks us to offer love, adoration and the sacrifice of our actions. In Bhakti Yoga our whole being has to be surrendered to the Spirit, and our entire consciousness raised up to dwell in the divine consciousness, so that the human Self can share in the Spirit's transcendence of nature and of actions. By doing this, we are able to act in life with a perfect spiritual liberty. We are free. And this freedom is yoga.

Understanding this mystical information, you can see my Divine power: whatever you sense or perceive in this world is that same power: and so you have yoga, the union with the divine. I am the source of everything: I am love. The yogis that give their minds and hearts fully to the Divine, know that God is the source of everything. With their attention and life energy flowing into me, absorbed in me, these yogis always speak of me with joy, and their lives are filled with peace and contentment. To those who are sincerely devoted and worship me simply out of love, I give them the yoga of vision, and with this they come to me.

Krishna tells Arjuna (and us):

You have been given the wisdom of yoga; listen to it, act on it and you can break through the bonds of karma. On this path, no effort made is lost and there are no adverse effects. Even a little practice of this dharma preserves one from fear. If your mind is chattering all the time and unsteady, there are too many choices and thoughts. But when your mind is clear and one-pointed, there is only one way to go.

And if we feel that this path is too hard, or the rewards seem too insubstantial, then we need to recall what all the yoga scriptures tell us are the results of practising yoga, even on the most obvious physical plane:

Perfection of our bodies means beauty, grace, strength, and being solid as a diamond.
When the yogi has full power over his body, he can increase the spiritual fire within, giving better health, a light body, and freedom from cravings.

The body of the person practising the regulation of breath becomes harmoniously developed, emits a sweet scent, and looks both beautiful and lovely.

The following qualities are surely always found in the body of every yogi: strong appetite, good digestion, cheerfulness, a handsome figure, great courage, mighty enthusiasm and full strength.

Not bad, eh?

15

The Last Word

As we age, life offers us countless opportunities to experience misery and suffering. Our bodies sag and droop from the effects of gravity, pains appear, and illnesses pay us unwanted and unwelcome visits. We feel time drawing away, casting us further and further from the shore, knowing that the time will one day arrive when we must drift completely away. But misery and suffering in old age don't have to be the only way to go. It is up to us how we perceive our old age, just as it is our own choice as to how we view all the earlier times of our life – childhood, youth and maturity.

The I Ching, the ancient Chinese oracle, says that in old age we must 'bang the drum and sing', defiantly and joyfully expressing the sheer pleasure of being, and the happiness of breathing, even when life itself is drawing to a close. If we choose to sit around and moan, instead of singing and drumming, then we will decline at an ever-increasing rate and finish our days drinking not the sweet wine of contentment, but the bitter tea of regret.

It is up to us to decide how we want to view the world: in misery, indifference or joy. The perception of our minds, the way we use our minds to see the world, determines whether we see everything as sacred and good, able to sustain and nourish us in loving relationships, or whether we see the world as a bleak uncaring place that we only inhabit for a short and fruitless time.

The freedom of the mind is our most precious freedom, since it allows us to create a world that we find congenial and satisfying, a world that reflects the goodness of the universe, and that shows us that whatever love we project and provide for others, returns to us in measureless ways. This is truly a miracle of existence, and one which yoga can lead us to.

The Buddhists ask, 'What is it that comes?' and by that they mean, what is it that you see approaching you in life, what is it that confronts you and happens to you, which you must deal with. That which comes at you is your Self, the feelings and thoughts that you have projected out into the world returning to you, just as a boomerang returns to the person who throws it. Our thoughts, speech and actions are like boomerangs that instantly, or gradually, or eventually return to us, and sometimes come back to haunt us. And if these thoughts and actions have been good, positive and loving, then the things that happen to us and appear to us will also be good and loving.

Evil exists, and evil can touch us and affect us, even when we have not been the originators of that evil. But as long as we do no evil, then we know in our deepest hearts that we have not been its cause, even though we may be touched by it. The Holocaust killed millions of people, many of whom were utterly saintly, pious and good, and who never harmed anyone. And yet they were indiscriminately killed, along with others who may have been less than saintly. Evil exists in the world, because people are capable of acting with the force of hatred and violence, but goodness also exists through the force of good and compassion, and it is our choice in life (indeed our task in life) to understand this, and to discover how best to make the choices that lead to co-operation, understanding and life, rather than the dark stench of evil and death.

I believe in the power of good to make a difference, and

I believe that those people who find a way to live with justice and compassion, for themselves and for others, reap rewards that are real, solid and everlasting, more important than the junk sold us by our consumerist culture.

Yoga is a path that leads to the freedom of the mind, and that freedom is our true freedom, an internal liberation that enables us to let go of harmful habits and compulsions that stifle our creativity in life, and expands the joy that results from expressing it. You may not follow this path to its ultimate end, but even to begin to walk this path can bring spiritual rewards that justify whatever time and effort you set aside for it. Yoga frees us from fear, and when fear is set aside, courage naturally arises, the courage to face the future without hesitation and apprehension, and the ability to live in the present with a feeling of absolute well-being. As my mother always said, 'There are some things money can't buy', and it is a truism that the best things in life are literally priceless.

After 40,000 words of trying to describe an experience that the yogis tell us requires only one word – OM – we would like to offer you some of Jo's thoughts on the crossover where philosophy and practice meet:

1. Do not strive, either in life or in yoga.
2. Be disciplined, but without using force: in breath, body, mind.
3. Your body is a temple housing your Spirit, treat it right, respect it, look after it.
4. The Spirit lives on after death, so individual achievement doesn't matter, as long as you find a connection to your Spirit during your lifetime.
5. Act with the heart and embody light and love.
6. Practise even when you feel lousy. When you practise, you come home to your body and to your breath, to

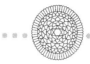

where you belong. 'Coming home' means connecting with the earth, and brings with it a sense of security and peace.

Returning to your mat is like returning home.

The final words. When I was at university I first read T. S. Eliot's poem, *The Waste Land*. I can't say that I understood much of it at the time, but I was always impressed with the ending of the poem, 'What the Thunder Said'. Researching for this book, I discovered that this section of Eliot's poem was taken from the *Brihadaranyaka Upanishad*, Brihadaranyaka meaning 'wisdom from the forest'. I'd like to end our introduction with this bit of forest teaching from the *Upanishad*, since I think it is something we need to hear again, and also because it sums up what I think is the true teaching of the yoga masters.

What the Thunder Said

The children of the Creator – gods, humans and the godless – all lived with Him as students.

When the gods had completed their studies, they said, 'Venerable One, Please teach us.'

The Creator answered with one syllable: **DA!**

'Do you understand?'

'Yes,' they said, 'you have told us to be self-controlled.'

'You have understood,' he said.

Next the human beings said, 'Venerable One, please teach us.'

The Creator answered again: **DA!**

'Do you understand?'

'Yes, you have told us to give.'

'You have understood.'

Then the godless approached. 'Venerable One, please teach us.'

The Creator said the same syllable: **DA!**

'Do you understand?'

'Yes, you have told us to be compassionate.'

'You have understood.'

The heavenly voice of thunder repeats this teaching:

DA!! DA!! DA!!
Be Self-controlled!
Give!
Be Compassionate!

OM Shanti Shanti Shanti
Let peace and peace and peace be everywhere

May the yogis of old, and the teachers of all the great spiritual traditions, from whose words we have learned wisdom and knowledge, bless the path you take and look after your wanderings, and may your personal God, even a God unknown to you, shine its light upon you, and bring you safely home to your heart.

Queens Park, London, June 2001–March 2002

PART TWO

Yoga's Sacred Scriptures

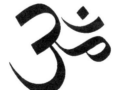

I

The Secret
Teachings

Selections from the Upanishads

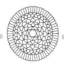

A Blessing

May we be blessed by the sun and the moon.
May we be blessed by the eye, strength, speech and space.
We welcome the Spirit, Life.
I shall only think truthful thoughts and speak truthful thoughts.
May truth protect my teacher and myself.
May we become illuminated with wisdom and united with the Spirit.

OM Shanti Shanti Shanti
May peace and peace and peace be everywhere.

TAITTIRIYA UPANISHAD

The Spirit Is with Us

The Universal Spirit exists in our hearts. Don't envy what others have, since we all belong to the same Spirit. If we can live with this feeling of Spirit in our hearts, we may live to be 100 years old. But even if we don't, our lives will be lived with a sense of freedom. Death is nothing to fear, because the Spirit is always with us.

The Spirit is everywhere. It moves away from us, yet remains within us. Without this Spirit, life could not exist. When we can see the Spirit in others, we feel no fear because we understand that we are all one. When we have this sense of unity, there is nothing to delude ourselves with, and we feel no sorrow or grief. We are all filled with the same light and innocence.

Meditate and pray that you may be filled with this light of the Universal Spirit. Trust in it, see it in all things and allow yourself to feel united with it. In this way, there is no evil, only good, and our hearts are full of love for ourselves and the world around us.

ISHA UPANISHAD

Spiritual Progress

What do we need?

To practise right conduct, learning and teaching. To be always honest, regulating our passions, controlling our senses, always striving for peace and serving humanity: this is what we must learn and teach. Learning and teaching are necessary for spiritual progress.

'I have become one with the tree of life. My glory is like a mountain peak. I have realized the Self, who is ever pure, wise, luminous and immortal,' said the sage Trishanku, attaining unity with the Lord of Love.

After explaining the scriptures, the teachers say, 'Speak the truth, do your duty. Don't neglect the scriptures. Give your best to your teacher, marry and continue the family. Don't neglect your spiritual or worldly welfare. Always learn and teach. Forget neither Spirit nor ancestor. See the Divine in your mother, father, teacher and guest. Never do what is wrong. Honour those who are worthy of honour. Give with faith and love and joy. If you are in doubt about the correct conduct, follow the advice of the sages as they know what is best for spiritual growth. This is the ancient teaching, this is the secret and the message.

TAITTIRIYA UPANISHAD

The Pure Mind

It is said that the mind can be both pure and impure. Driven by the senses, it becomes impure, but with the senses under control, the mind can become pure. It is the mind that frees us or enslaves us. When we are driven by the senses we become bound; if we seek freedom we must master our senses.

When the mind is detached from the senses we reach the height of awareness. Mastery of the mind leads to wisdom. We must practice meditation and stop all vain chatter. The highest state is beyond our thoughts.

Keep repeating the ancient mantra OM until it reverberates in your heart. Brahman, the Supreme Spirit, is indivisible and pure; when we realize the Eternal Spirit we go beyond all change. This Spirit is immanent and transcendent. Sages have said that when they realize Him there are no separate minds, but they realize who they always are. Waking, sleeping, dreaming, the Self is One. Transcend these states and go beyond rebirth.

There is only one Self in all creatures. The One appears many, just as the moon appears as many when it is reflected in water. The Self appears to change its location but does not, just as the air in a jar does not change when the jar is transported. The air doesn't know when the jar is broken, but the Self knows when the body dies.

We cannot see ourselves when we are concealed by illusion, but when the veil of illusion falls we can see the Self.

Repeating OM, the symbol of the Eternal Spirit, can bring peace to the mind.

Knowledge is twofold, lower and higher. Realize the Self, for all else is lower: realization is the rice; all else is chaff. The sages say that wisdom is the milk and the sacred scriptures are the cows.

As butter lies hidden within milk, the Self is hidden in our hearts. Churn the mind in meditation on it; light your fire through meditation on it: the Self – all whole, all peace, all certainty.

The sage declares, 'I have realized the Self who is present in all beings, and I am united with the Lord of Love.'

Amritabindu Upanishad

The Enlightened One

Narada asked the Lord of Love, 'What is the state of the enlightened person?'

The Lord replied, 'It is very hard to reach that state, and only few attain it; but even one is enough. She who is enlightened is truly great, because she serves me and I reveal myself through her always.

'She has renounced all selfish attachments and observes no rites and ceremonies. She has minimal possessions and lives her life for the good of all humanity.

'She faces heat and cold, pleasure and pain, honour and dishonour with equal calm; she is not affected by pride, jealousy, status, joy or sorrow, greed, anger or infatuation, excitement or egoism; for she knows she is neither body nor mind.

'Free from the sway of doubt and false knowledge, she lives united with the Lord of Love who is ever serene, immutable, the source of all joy and wisdom. The Lord of Love is her true home, for she has entered the integrated state.

'Having renounced every selfish desire, she has found her rest in the Lord of Love. When we are at the mercy of our senses we cannot escape enormous suffering; the enlightened person knows this to be the truth of life. For her the universe is her clothing, and the Lord is not separate from her. She praises no one, blames no one and is never dependent on anyone. She sees God in all.

'When we seek the Lord of Love we must free ourselves from selfish attachments to people, money and possessions. When our minds have shed every selfish desire we are able to rule our senses. Then we will not bear ill will to anyone; we will no longer be in a state of elation, for our senses will be stilled and will come to rest in our Self, entering an integrated state. This is the goal of evolution.'

Parahamsa Upanishad

Inner Peace

When you become wise and reach the state of union with your inner Self, desiring nothing in the physical world, you become one with the Lord of Love. But if you let your mind wander among your desires, longing for objects of desire, you will live in a world of separateness disconnected from your true Self. When you realize that you are in fact your inner Self, you will find that union. This does not come from talking or from your intellect, nor from the study of the scriptures. This inner connection can only come to you if you long with all your heart to be connected to your Self, your inner Spirit.

We cannot find our Self if we are weak or careless, or if we practise the wrong disciplines. It can only come to us when we are pure and truthful.

What the sages in their devotion to the Lord of Love have been looking for they have found at last: inner peace. Seeing the Lord of Love everywhere and in everything, they are united with Him forever. They have reached the highest spiritual place and have reached immortality. When their bodies die, their life force returns to a cosmic womb, but their work in life brings others together with their inner Self.

As the rivers flow into the ocean to find their final peace, and their names and forms disappear, so the wise become free from their names and forms, and become one with the Supreme Spirit.

This wisdom should only be taught to those who follow the law of life's unity and offer their lives to the Lord of Love. In truth, those who know the Eternal Self become the Eternal Spirit.

MUNDAKA UPANISHAD

Yoga Cleanses the Spirit

May we harness our bodies and minds to see the Lord of Life who dwells in everyone.

May we maintain a one-pointed mind striving for a blissful union with the Lord.

May we train our senses to serve the Lord through the practice of meditation.

Kindle the fire of your life force and your spirit deep in meditation. Bring your mind and your breath under control. Allow yourself to feel deeply a sense of Divine love and you will attain the state of union of body, spirit and mind. Dedicate yourself to the Lord of Life and you will be purified of your past sins and become free from the bondage of karma.

Sit with your spine erect and lead your mind and your senses inward; use the mantra OM and let it echo in your heart, freeing you from fear and sorrow. When your body becomes silent and steady, breathing rhythmically through the nose, you can train your senses to be quiet. The chariot of the mind is drawn by wild horses and those wild horses have to be tamed.

Choose a clean, quiet and cool place for meditation and the practice of yoga, where the sounds of dancing water and the beauty of the place foster thought and contemplation. In deep meditation you may see forms like snow or smoke, you may feel a strong wind blowing, or a wave of heat, or you may see more and more light within. These are signs that you are on the spiritual path to reach the Eternal Spirit of Brahman.

When the yogi has full power over his body, he can increase the spiritual fire within, giving better health, a light body and freedom from craving. When a gold mirror is covered with dust, it shines again when it has been cleaned. When you have been cleansed with the truth of the Spirit your life is fulfilled and you are beyond suffering. Then you become a lamp by which you find the truth of the Spirit and see the pure Everlasting Spirit, freeing you from all bondage.

This is the Spirit whose light illumines all Creation, the Creator of all from the beginning. He was, He is and always shall be; He is in all and sees all. Let us adore the Lord of Life who is ever present in fire, water, plants and trees.

SHVETASHVATARA UPANISHAD

The Ocean of Existence

In the beginning, there was only one Self. He thought, 'Let me create the world,' and He did. He created all the worlds: those of earth, light and water. He thought to himself, 'I have created these worlds, now let me create guardians for these worlds.' He lifted an egg from the water. He warmed it and, because of His warmth, a being with a mouth appeared through a crack in the shell. From the mouth came speech; from speech came fire. Then nostrils appeared with the power to breathe the air, eyes opened giving rise to sight and the sun, and ears opened to hear the sounds of the universe. Then skin appeared and from that, hair; from hair came plants and trees. The heart appeared, and from the heart came the mind, and from the mind came the moon. The navel opened with the downward force of the breath of apana, giving rise to death. The sexual organ appeared, and from this organ came seed and from seed, water – giving rise to birth.

This is how these guardians came into the mighty ocean of existence. The Self then caused them to feel hunger and thirst. They said to the Self, 'Give us a place where we can live and eat.' The Self brought them a cow, but they said, 'This is not what we desire.' So He brought them a horse, but again they said, 'This is not what we desire.' Then He brought them a human form and they said in joy, 'This is perfect, the human body is exactly right for us. The Self asked them to enter the body and take up their places. Fire becoming speech entered the mouth; air becoming smell entered the nose; the sun becoming sight entered the eyes; the sounds of the universe becoming hearing entered the ears; plants becoming hair entered the skin; the moon becoming mind entered the heart; the God of Death becoming the downward force entered the navel; the God of Living Water becoming sperm entered the sex organ.

Finally hunger and thirst said to the Self, 'Give us a place to live.' He told them, 'Enter these guardians and share their life with them.' So now, whatever we do in life, we can feel hunger, thirst and pleasure.

The Self, the Creator, thought, 'Here are the worlds and their guardians. I need to create food for them.' He meditated on water and from the heat of meditation came an image, and that image was food. Food tried to run away from man in fear.

Man tried to catch it with speech, but he couldn't because merely saying the name of food doesn't satisfy hunger.

He tried to catch it with his breath, but couldn't because smelling the food doesn't satisfy hunger.

He tried to catch it with his eyes, but couldn't because looking at food doesn't satisfy hunger.

He tried to catch it with his ears, but couldn't because hearing about food doesn't satisfy hunger.

He tried to catch it with his skin, but couldn't because touching food doesn't satisfy hunger.

He tried to catch it with his mind but couldn't because thinking about food doesn't satisfy hunger.

He tried to catch it with his genitalia, but couldn't because sexual union doesn't satisfy hunger.

He tried to catch it with the downward force of the apana breath and at last he caught it.

Thus it is that the downward energy of digestion takes in food and lives on food.

The Self thought, 'If speaking is done by speech, breathing by breath, seeing by eyes, hearing by ears, smelling by nose and meditation by the mind, then who am I? Can they live without me? How shall I enter the body?' So He entered the body through the gateway at the crown of the head. He found three places in the body where He could live, three states where He could move: in waking, dreaming and sleeping. As He entered the body He wondered if there could be anything in the body that was not Himself, and He was happy to find that there was nothing but Himself.

AITAREYA UPANISHAD

The Universal Spirit

The student asks, 'Where do my thoughts come from? How did my life begin? Where do my words come from? Who is this God, this Universal Spirit who sees through my eyes, and hears through my ears?'

The teacher replies, 'It is the Universal Spirit that exists in all that lives. If we can rise above our senses and our conscious mind and realize that we are really one with all beings, we become immortal. We have heard wise enlightened beings say that there are no answers to be found other than within ourselves. This Universal Spirit is none other than you.

'If you think you know this Universal Spirit, then you really don't because what you know is only your subjective mind. So you must keep meditating.'

The student says, 'I can't really say if I know Him or not.'

The teacher answers, 'If we believe we know, we don't. If we believe we don't know, we probably do. It's a mistake to think that we know what this Universal Spirit is from intellectual understanding; it is beyond knowledge. When we have reached a deep state of meditation, we overcome the thoughts that tell us that we are a body that is born and will die, and are able to connect ourselves to the Universal Spirit that goes beyond death. If we find that higher power, we find the ultimate truth, but if not we live in darkness and fear.'

When we forget that we are part of the Universal Spirit and find our minds thinking about things we desire, feeling anger, hatred or other negative emotions, and try to will life to be the way we want it to be, we have to come back to our meditation. It is through this meditation and connection to the higher powers of life that we find peace, acceptance and love – love for ourselves, love for others and an intimate connection to all living things. It is only through meditation and prayer that we can live in selfless service to the world and understand the truth of the universe.

Kena Upanishad

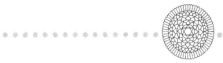

The Deathless Spirit

The Creator came first, having created Himself. He called Himself the Protector of the world. He passed on to His eldest son Atharva the knowledge of Spirit, which is the foundation of all wisdom. Atharva gave it to Angi, who in turn gave it to Satyavaha, who in succession passed it on to Angiras.

One day a man called Shaunaka approached Angiras reverently and asked, 'Master, what is it that allows us to know everything in the world?'

Angiras replied, 'Sages say that there are two kinds of wisdom, the higher and the lower. Lower knowledge is understood as the study of the scriptures, linguistics and astronomy. Higher wisdom is known as Self-realization, an understanding of the Everlasting Spirit. The Spirit cannot be seen, nor can the mind grasp it. The Deathless Spirit has no caste or race; it has no eyes, hands or feet. Sages say that this Spirit is infinite in both the great and the small, prevalent everywhere and always alive. The sages say that our universe springs from the Deathless Spirit, the source of life.'

Just as the spider weaves his web and then withdraws, as plants sprout from the soil, and hair grows from the body, so our universe springs from the Deathless Spirit, the source of life.

Through the power of meditation, the Deathless Spirit created the universe as evolutionary energy; from this energy life, the mind and the elements all developed, as did the world of karma, the chain of cause and effect.

The Creator, embodying the process of evolution into name and form, comes from the Deathless Spirit, who sees all and knows all.

MUNDAKA UPANISHAD

Lower and Higher Knowledge

The rituals and sacrifices described in the scriptures deal with lower knowledge. The sages ignored these rituals and sought higher knowledge. But if you seek rewards for your actions, then stay with the rituals. If you follow the path of higher knowledge, you will shine in the light of the Creator. If you follow the rituals inappropriately and are ignorant of your ignorance, then you will find the crossing of the sea of sorrow rough going, and you will follow the difficult path of your karma. This happens when fools think themselves wise and go through life like the blind leading the blind. The proud think they have solved every problem while the passionate never learn, so they find themselves thrust from paradise into the misery of life.

But those that are pure in heart, who practise meditation and are able to still their senses and passions, become immortal and connect to their inner essence. This inner essence is their Self and is the source of all light and the source of all life. Those that understand the Law of Karma do not perform bad deeds. So understand that if you are seeking pleasure or profit, you will never cross the sea of sorrow. Find a teacher who has found her inner essence, her true Self. She can reveal the Lord of Love to a student whose heart is full of love, and whose mind and senses are at peace.

MUNDAKA UPANISHAD

The Four Questions

What is this world? The earth is below, the sky is above, there is air between and space joining them.

What are the other heavenly bodies? Fire is on one side

and the sun on the other, there is water between and lightning connects them.

What is education? Teacher on one side, pupil on the
other, knowledge between them and discussion joins them.

What is generation? Mother on one side, father on the
other, the child between, and procreation joins them.

The one who knows this will have children, cattle, food
and wisdom.

TAITTIRIYA UPANISHAD

The Eternal Questions

What is the source of the universe? What is the Eternal Spirit
we call Brahman? Where do we come from? By what power
do we live? Where do we find peace? Who rules over our joys
and our sorrows?

We could think about time, or the nature of things, or the
law of necessity, or of chance, or of the elements, or of the
power of creation of woman or man. These are only effects
whose purpose is to help the Self rise above pleasure and
pain. The sages in the depths of meditation see the power of
the Lord of Love hidden in his own Creation. He dwells deep
in the heart of every creature, hidden behind the three forces
of Nature: harmony, activity and inertia. He is One, and rules
over time, space and causality.

The world is the wheel of God turning around and
around with all living creatures clinging to its rim. The world
is the river of God, flowing from Him and back to Him. The
individual Self goes around and around on this constantly
revolving wheel of being, through life after life, believing
himself to be a separate creature. When the Lord of Love
comes down upon us, then we find our own immortal life.

The Lord of Love holds the world in His hands: this

universe composed of the changing and the changeless, the transient and the eternal, the seen and the unseen. The human Self is bound by pleasure and pain but when she sees God she is liberated.

Conscious Spirit and unconscious Matter have existed since the dawn of time, with illusion, maya, appearing to connect them, misrepresenting joy as outside us. When we see all these as one, the Self reveals his universal form and serves as an instrument of the Divine will.

Meditate on God because through contemplating Him and by communing with Him, we can reach the end of the destructive earthly delusion. When we know God we are free. When we no longer identify ourselves with our bodies we can go beyond birth and death. We find the world of the Spirit where the power of the All is, and we have it all. For we are one with the ONE.

Know that the Eternal Spirit Brahman is always inside our hearts. Really and truly there is nothing more to know in this life. Meditate and realize that this world is filled with the presence of God.

Fire is hidden in matches, and we do not see it until a match is struck. Just as oil is hidden in sesame seeds, and butter hidden in cream, in the same way the Lord of Love is hidden in our hearts, until we realize him through truth and meditation. Realize the Self in the depths of meditation, who is the Lord of Love, the supreme Reality that is the goal of all knowledge. This is the highest mystical teaching.

SHVETASHVATARA UPANISHAD

God Is Pure Consciousness

Some learned people say that life is self-created; others say that life has evolved over time. It is the Lord who has brought the cosmos out of Himself.

The whole universe is always in His power. He is pure consciousness, the Creator of time, all-powerful, all-knowing and master of the three forces of Nature.

When we act without any desire for personal profit and lead a well-disciplined life we discover in the course of time that all forms of life are one. When we work in the service of the Lord we are freed from the Law of Karma.

Deep in meditation we may see Him, knowing that He is the primal source of life whose glory permeates the universe. He is the supreme Lord of Lords, king of kings, God of gods, ruler of all, without action or organs of action, whose power is seen in every way. We cannot see how He works or what tools He uses. There is nothing that we can compare with Him, since nothing is greater than Him. His power is shown in so many ways; His work and wisdom are great. There was no one before Him, and no one rules over Him because He is the source of all and the ruler of all. May God who is hidden in nature, even as the silkworm is hidden in the web of silk, lead us to union with His own Spirit, Brahman. The Lord of Love hidden in the innermost soul of all beings watches over the works of Creation.

The Lord is the operator and we are His innumerable instruments. May we in our consciousness realize the bliss that He alone can give us. Changeless amidst the changing, consciousness of the conscious, He grants all our prayers. May we in our consciousness realize the freedom that He alone can give us.

The sun, moon and stars do not shine, but everything reflects the light of the Lord. His radiance illuminates all Creation. He is the everlasting wandering swan, the soul of all in the universe, the spirit of fire in the ocean of life. To know Him is to overcome death and He is the only path to life eternal.

Longing for liberation, we must go for refuge to God who is one in the silence of eternity, pure radiance of beauty and perfection. This is where we find our peace. He is the supreme bridge that leads us to immortality and the spirit of fire burning away all the dross of our lives.

If it were ever possible to fold up the sky like a piece of material, we might be able to end our sorrow without His help.

The sage Shvetashvatara realized the Lord of Love in meditation and then imparted this sacred wisdom to his devoted disciples. If you have a deep love for the Lord of Love and for your teacher, the light of this teaching will shine in your heart: it shines in a great soul.

SHVETASHVATARA UPANISHAD

As Above, So Below

The sage contemplated the outer elements of earth, sun, fire and water, and the inner elements of eye, ear, mind, bones, skin and muscles and he discovered . . . everything is holy! With the help of the outer elements, one can regulate the inner elements.

TAITTIRIYA UPANISHAD

The Spiritual Seekers

Part One: The Creator

Sukesha, Satyakama, Gargya, Kausalya, Bhargava and Kabandhi were students filled with devotion for the Eternal Spirit. They decided one day that the holy guru Pippalada could explain to them all the sacred teachings for Self-realization. So they decided to approach him for his guidance on the spiritual path.

The sage told them that if they lived with him for a year,

practising meditation to control the senses and to find ultimate trust in the universe, then they could ask whatever they wanted, and he would answer them.

All agreed and when the year ended, Kabandhi asked the sage, 'Master, who created the universe?'

The Sage replied, 'In the beginning, the Creator longed for the joy of Creation. He meditated for a long time and then he found prana, the breath of life energy, and also rayi, matter.' He thought, these two, prana and rayi, male and female, will produce beings for me. The sun is life, the moon is matter. All that has form, solid or subtle, is matter: therefore form is matter. The sun gives light and life to all who live, and is the life energy of the universe.

'Therefore, the wise see the Lord of Love in the sun rising in its golden radiance to give warmth, light and love to all.

'The year is the Creator. There are two paths, the way of the south and the way of the north. Those who think that they have performed sacrifices and done pious work only get to the region of the moon and return to life and death. That is why those sages who desire children and the life of the family follow the path of the South. This is the path that leads to the ancestors.

'But those who are in search of the inner Spirit follow the spiritual path of the north with steadiness, purity, faith and wisdom. It is they who find the solar world, which is living, immortal and beyond fear: this is the goal. Once there, they do not return.

'Some look upon the sun as our father of the north, who makes life possible with heat and rain, and divides time into months and seasons. Others speak of a sage in the south with a chariot of seven colours as His seven horses, and six spinning wheels to represent the whirling spokes of time.

'The wise see the Lord of Love in the month: rayi, matter, is the dark half of the moon's phase, and prana is the bright.

The wise worship in the light of wisdom while others linger in the darkness of ignorance.

'The wise also see the Lord of Love as each day. Rayi, matter, is the dark night, while prana, life energy, is daylight. Those who use their days for sexual pleasure consume their prana, the very essence of life; but when mastered and used at night, sexuality becomes a highly spiritual force.

'The wise see the Lord of Love in all food. From food comes seed, and from seed all creatures. Those who live to fulfil sexual desires take the lunar path, but those who are self-regulated, pure and truthful, will go to the bright regions of the sun.'

Part Two: The Powers

Next Bhargava asked the sage, 'What powers have knitted the body together? What powers give it life, and which is the greatest of these?'

The sage responded, 'The powers are air, fire, water, earth, speech, mind, sight and hearing. These powers believed that it was they together who kept the union of the person, and are its foundation.

'But prana, life energy, the power supreme, said to them, 'Do not deceive yourselves. It is I alone who hold this body together.' But the powers did not believe him.

'To demonstrate the truth, prana rose and left the body and with the life energy drained, all the powers understood that they too had to leave. When prana agreed to return to the body, they too came back. Just as bees follow their queen when she goes out and return when she returns, speech, mind, sight and hearing returned. The powers then understood the truth and joyfully sang this song of life:

"Prana, life, is the fire that burns and is the sun that gives light. Life is the wind and the rain and the thunder in the sky. Life is matter and earth, what is and what is not, and what is beyond, in eternity. Everything is fixed in life, as the spokes of a wheel are fixed into the hub: all the sacred scriptures, all the rituals, all the warriors and kings. You, the Lord of Creation, who enters the womb of the mother as life to be manifested again, are honoured by all creatures. You, the Lord of Creation, who give gifts to the gods and the fathers, and help sages master their senses, which depend upon you for their function. You are the Creator, destroyer, and our protector. You shine as the sun in the sky: you are the source of all light. When you pour yourself down as rain on the earth, every living creature is filled with joy and knows that food will be abundant for all. You are pure and master of everything. It is you who gives us the breath of life. Be kind to us with your invisible form, be with us in sight, speech, hearing and mind and don't abandon us. Oh prana, the whole world depends on you as a mother looks after her children. Look after us and grant us happiness and wisdom."'

Part Three: Prana Is Life

Then the student Kausalya asked the sage, 'Lord, when does life begin? How does it get into the body? How does it live there? How does it leave the body when the body dies? How does it support all that is outside and all that is inside?'

The sage replied, 'You ask heavy questions, digging deep into the root of life. Since you are a devoted seeker, I will answer you. Life, prana, comes from the Self. At the time of birth, the Self puts life into the body so that the mind's desires can be fulfilled. In the same way that a king appoints officials to rule certain cities on his behalf, so prana, the ruler of life, rules the other living powers of the body. Apana, the energy of exhalation, rules the sexual organs and excretion. Prana lives in the eyes and the ears and moves through the nose and the mouth. Samana, the life force that nourishes the body by digesting and distributing food, and lighting up the seven bodily functions, is located in the middle of the body. Radiating from the heart where your Self dwells, vyana, the distributor of energy, moves through the myriad of vital currents. Udana, the fifth energy force, leads the man of good actions to reward and the man of evil actions to punishment.

'The rising sun is the symbol of life; it rises to bring light to our eyes. The earth draws the lower fire of apana; the space between sun and earth is samana and the moving air is vyana. Udana is the fire inside. When that fire goes out, the senses are drawn back into the mind and the person is ready for rebirth. A person's last thoughts before death lead him to prana, and accompanied by the living fire of udana, the individual Self is led to be reborn in the place it has earned.

'The person who understands the meaning of life goes beyond death, and his children are never lost. He who knows the source and power of life, how it enters, where it lives, how it works, and how it is related to the true Self within, attains immortality.'

Part Four: The Self

Then Gargya approached the sage and asked him, 'Sir, when someone sleeps, who is it that sleeps in him? What power is it that sees his dreams? When he wakes up, what is it in him that is awake? Who experiences the happiness? On what do all these depend?'

The sage replied, 'In the same way that the rays of the sun become one with the sphere of the sun at the end of the day, before they spread out again at sunrise, so the senses gather themselves up into the mind, master of them all.

Therefore when a person neither hears, sees, smells, tastes, touches, speaks nor enjoys, we say he sleeps.

'But in the city of the body, the fires of life are burning – they never sleep. Apana is like a sacred home fire forever kept burning from father to son. Vyana is like the fire of the south for offerings to the ancestors. Prana, the life energy, is like the fire of the east lit up by the home fire. Samana is the equalizing fire that balances the inbreath and the outbreath. Udana is the fruit of dreamless sleep in which the mind is led close to the true Self within.

'The dreaming mind recalls past impressions. What it has seen it sees again, what it has heard, it hears again, what it has enjoyed in different countries and climates, it enjoys again. The mind knows everything, things that have been seen and unseen, heard and unheard, felt and not felt, real and unreal. When the mind is stilled in a deep and dreamless sleep, the body rests deeply and finds joy and peace.

'Just as birds fly to their tree for rest, all living things find rest in their Self. The earth, water, fire, air, space as well as sight, hearing, smell, taste, and touch all find their final peace in their inner Self. So too does the voice, the hands, and all powers of action, the mind and what it thinks, the intellect and what it knows, the ego and what it grasps, the heart and what it loves, the light and what it reveals: all things find their rest in the spirit when they are in dreamless sleep.

'It is one's inner Self who sees, hears, smells, touches, tastes, thinks, acts and is pure awareness; and one's Self finds peace in the eternal and Supreme Spirit, Brahman. The Personal Self and the Impersonal Spirit are one. Those who know the Eternal Spirit as formless, without shadow, without impurity, know all and live in all. Those who know the individual Self, the seat of all consciousness, in whom the breath and the senses live, know all and live in all.

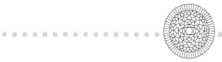

Part Five: OM

The disciple Satyakama asked, 'If someone meditated until his death on OM, what would happen to him?'

The sage responded, 'The word OM is both the transcendent and the immanent highest spiritual power. By chanting this sacred word, the wise connect to this highest power.

'OM has three sounds – A,U, M. Those that meditate on the first sound – A – will be born again on this earth to lead a pure life, full of love and faith. Those who meditate on the first two sounds – A and U – go to the lunar world, and after enjoying their heavenly joys, come back to earth again. But if, by meditating on the three sounds of the eternal OM – A,U, M, the wise person puts his mind in meditation upon the Supreme Spirit, he enters the regions of the full light of the sun, where he is freed from all evil and is connected to the highest Spirit.

'If the three sounds are not used together, you are led again to life that dies. When the whole mantra – A, U and M – are used together indivisible and interdependent, the sound reverberates in the mind and, whether awake or asleep, one is freed from fear, and enters into infinite peace.'

Part Six: Realize The Self

Now Sukesha said, 'Master, the Prince of Kosala asked me once if I knew the Self and its sixteen forms. I told him that I didn't, but that if I did I would have told him. I said that if I was lying to him, I should wither like a tree to its roots: I did not want to be untruthful. The Prince remained silent, mounted his chariot and rode away. Now may I ask you, where is that Eternal Self?'

The sage replied, 'Oh my son, the Self with its sixteen

forms is here within your body. The Self asked Himself what it was that drove Him to go when He goes, and stay when He stays. So He created prana, the life energy, and from prana, desire; from desire He made space, wind, light, water and earth. From the earth He made the senses, and from the senses the mind. Finally, He created food, and from food came strength, discipline, the scriptures, sacrifice and all the worlds, and everything was given a name and a form.

'When rivers flow towards the ocean they find their final peace, and they are no longer known as rivers once they become part of the ocean. In the same way all the sixteen forms disappear when the Self is realized. Then we no longer have a name or a form and we attain immortality.'

The sage concluded, 'Up to now, I know the Supreme Self and there is nothing beyond that.'

The students bowed to the teacher in adoration and said, 'You are our true teacher who has taken us from ignorance and led us on our spiritual journey to the other shore across the sea.'

PRASHNA UPANISHAD

All Is OM

OM is Spirit. Everything is OM. OM is the beginning of the ancient chants. The priests start with OM, the teachers start with OM. The student murmuring OM seeks the Spirit and finds it in the end.

TAITTIRIYA UPANISHAD

The Word

Let us meditate on OM, the beginning of prayer.

The essence of all beings is the earth; the essence of the

earth is water; the essence of water is plants; the essence of plants, the human; the essence of the human, speech; and the essence of speech is OM.

OM represents the highest Spirit, so it is the essence of essences, that which we humans take as being holy. At the heart of prayer, like a couple coming together to fulfil each other's desire, speech and breath come together as the imperishable OM. When we meditate on OM, our desires are fulfilled. With the word OM we say 'I agree' and fulfil desires. When we chant OM, we honour the sounds of the word which is the key to knowledge and the higher Spirit, which we call Brahman.

When we simply make the sound of OM as a recitation, and when we chant the sound of OM with its meaning understood, it would seem that we are doing the same thing. However, when we chant OM with knowledge, inner awareness and faith, we grow in power.

CHANDOGYA UPANISHAD

The Four States of Consciousness

The sound OM represents the Supreme Reality of the visible and invisible universe. Past, present and future – everything is OM, and whatever goes beyond what was, what is and what shall be is also this sound – OM. All is OM.

There is nothing that is not Spirit. Your inner Self is also Spirit, self-same, identical, and it exists in four states.

The first is the waking life, called Vaishvanara, when our consciousness turns outward through the senses, focused only on the material world.

The second is the dreaming state, Taijasa, the shining one, when our senses are turned inward, and we re-enact the subtle and luminous impressions of past deeds, present desires and fears of the future.

The third is deep sleep, Prajna, the all-knowing, when there are neither dreams nor desires. The mind switches off in Prajna, and there is no experience of separateness, but the sleeper is unaware of this. When the sleeper can become conscious while in Prajna, the door to peace and joy opens.

The fourth condition is super-consciousness, called Turiya, pure awareness, when a person is neither inward nor outward, and is beyond the senses and the intellect: he is in fact nothing more than the individual Real Self, Atman. He realizes the supreme goal of life: infinite peace and love. Realize your true Self, the peaceful, blissful Atman.

The state of Turiya, the Real Self, is represented by OM. Though OM is indivisible it has three sounds – A, U and M – corresponding to the first three states of the Self.

The first sound – A – is the first state of waking consciousness, common to us all. The letter A leads off the alphabet and breathes in all the other letters. When you understand this you obtain all you want and can become a leader.

The dreaming state corresponds to the second letter – U. Those that know this by mastering even their dreams, become wise and attain equilibrium.

Dreamless sleep corresponds to the third letter – M. Those that understand this and can still their minds find their true stature, and inspire everyone around them to grow.

The word OM as one indivisible sound is the fourth state of supreme consciousness, a silence and wholeness beyond birth and death, the symbol of everlasting joy. Those that know OM as the inner Self become the Impersonal Self, the Spirit, so OM is nothing but eternal intermingled Self and Spirit.

MANDUKYA UPANISHAD

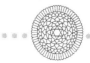

The Self Lies Hidden in the Heart

Bright but hidden, the Self dwells in the heart. Everything that moves and breathes lives in the Self. He is the source of love and can only be found with real and pure love, but not with thought. The Lord of Love is the goal for our lives. Walk this spiritual path and find Him.

The shining Self dwells deep in the heart. Everything in the world lives in the Self. The Lord of Love is the source of life and truth.

Consider sacred knowledge as a bow, and your soul as an arrow; then draw the bowstring of meditation and aim at the target to become one with the Lord of Love. The sky, earth and air are all woven in Him. Get to know Him as the one and only, the bridge to immortality. Do not speak in vain.

He is in the centre of your being. Meditate on the sound of OM, knowing that therein lies the Lord of Love. May His blessing take you out of darkness.

The Lord of Love knows all and sees all. Based deep in your heart, He guides body and life. Finding Him brings you peace, joy, light and life eternal. When we truly connect to Him in our hearts, all our doubts and pains from past actions are released. Know the Lord of Love as the radiant light of lights. He lights the sun, moon and stars and his radiance illuminates all creation. The eternal spirit is everywhere, to the left of you, to the right of you, above and below, in front and behind. What is this world but Spirit?

Mundaka Upanishad

Two Golden Birds

Like two intimate friends, two golden birds perch on the same tree. One eats the tree's fruit, while the other looks on in peaceful and detached silence. The first bird is the ego, who eventually gets tired of pecking here and there and becomes dejected, just as we do when we are attached to things. However, when we realize that we are really the second bird, the Self, the Lord of Life, and meditate on this, we free ourselves from suffering. When we realize that we are the true Self, the Spirit, the source of light and love, then we meet yoga in its true sense: the union of spirit, body and mind.

The Lord of Love shines in everyone's heart. When we are wise and see the Lord of Love in all living things, we lose ourselves in the service of all and find ultimate peace and joy. With truth, meditation, self-control and discipline, we find ourselves in this state of joy and see the inner spirit, our real essence, shining in our hearts.

To be truthful is the right way, and the way to this truth is to live without desire. Truth lies beyond imagination, beyond paradise. Truth lies in the inmost centre of the heart. Truth is beyond the reach of the senses and can be reached through the practice of deep meditation, where the mind is pure and still.

When you are pure in mind and spirit, you get what you want: a life of joy and peace.

MUNDAKA UPANISHAD

Self and Spirit Are One

In the same way that thousands of sparks come from a fire and go back into the fire, so an infinity of beings are given life by the Creator, the Lord of Love, and return to Him.

This everlasting Lord of Love is shapeless, unborn, breathless, without body or mind, above everything, outside everything, and yet inside everything. From Him comes life and mind and the senses of all life. From Him comes space and light, air, fire and water and this earth that supports us all.

The Lord of Love is the innermost Self of all. His head

relates to fire, His eyes to the sun and moon; His ears relate to heaven, and the sacred scriptures to His voice; the air relates to His breath, the universe to His heart, and the earth to His footrest.

From Him comes the fire that burns in the sky; this fire fuels the sun, from the sun comes the moon, the rain descends because of the moon, food arises from rain, man lives on food, and seed comes from man; so you see that everything descends from the Lord of Love.

There is nothing in this world that is not the Lord of Love. He is action, purity, everlasting spirit. From Him comes all the scripture and rituals. From Him spring the gods of the natural world, men, beasts, birds and the food that nourishes them. From Him come all spiritual disciplines, meditation, truth, faith, and purity. From Him come all the seas and the mountains, the rivers and the plants that support life. He dwells in the heart as the innermost Self of all.

The Lord of Love is the one Self of all. He is spiritual wisdom and immortality. Find your innermost Spirit and stop being ignorant.

MUNDAKA UPANISHAD

The Seventh Chakra

The Lord of Love lives deep in the heart, filling it with immortality, light and wisdom. Locate the uppermost chakra at the top of the skull and chant 'maha' with the vibration of that energy centre. This will allow you to become king of your own life, ruler of your passions, senses and intellect. When you unite with the Lord of Love, you become the Spirit itself in truth, peace and immortality. Meditate always on the Lord of Love and you will live with the source of joy, the supreme goal of life.

TAITTIRIYA UPANISHAD

A Dialogue with Death

Part One: The Sacrifice

Once, long ago, there was a man called Vajasravasa who so desired heavenly approval that he gave away many of his possessions as a sacrifice to the Gods. He had a son called Nachiketa who, though young, had diligently studied the scriptures. When his father made his offerings Nachiketa wondered what his father gained by sacrificing old dried-up cows too weak to eat grass or drink water. Nachiketas wanted his father to see that giving up something that had no further use to him was not much of a sacrifice, so he asked his father whether there was anything that he would sacrifice his own son for. His father didn't want to respond, but Nachiketa kept nagging at him, until his father finally responded angrily that he would sacrifice Nachiketa for death.

Nachiketa asked himself what difference it would make if he died now or later, since, like everyone else, he was bound, eventually, to die. What really interested him would be to meet the God of Death now, while he was still alive.

Vajasravasa, on hearing his son's thoughts, wanted to retract his words, but Nachiketa said to him, 'Think of all those who have died and all those that will die. Man is born, dies and then is born again, just like a head of corn.'

So Nachiketa went into the forest to visit the House of Death. Not finding Death at home, he sat down and meditated for three days without eating. When Death finally appeared, Nachiketa's servant asked Death to give his guest water, and to receive the holy man well.

Death said to Nachiketa, 'I will give you three gifts to repay you for the three inhospitable nights you have spent waiting for me.'

Nachiketa thought this over and responded, 'As my first

gift, I would like my father to be free of anger and to welcome me back in peace and love.'

Death said, 'I will arrange that when you return and your father sees that you have been released from the jaws of Death, he will sleep peacefully again and welcome you back with open arms.'

Nachiketa was pleased with this, so he said, 'As my second gift, I would like you to teach me about the fire of sacrifice. We know that in heaven there is no such thing as fear of old age or death since you, Death, are not there, so we rejoice in the kingdom of heaven which lies beyond hunger, thirst or sorrow.'

Death answered, 'Of course I know about the fire of life and I will agree to teach it to you.'

So Death explained the fire of creation and how to build the altar, showing Nachiketa how many bricks to use and where to place them. When Nachiketa repeated the instructions he had been given, Death was pleased and said:

'I am going to give you a special gift; this fire shall be named after you. And I will give you a further gift of a chain; it is the chain of those who light the fire three times, connecting themselves to the mother, father and teacher. Those who perform the three duties of study, sacrifice and charity pass beyond life, death and sorrow and find joy in heaven. When a person understands the essence of Self, and also understands the Universal Spirit, the union of these two kindles this triple fire and offers the sacrifice. Then one can live without fear of death and without sorrow. Now, what is your third request?'

Nachiketa said, 'Some people say that when you die you are nothing, while others say you still exist. Which of these is true?'

Death replied, 'This is a very difficult question, which the Gods have discussed endlessly. Please ask me something else.'

But Nachiketa was not easily put off. 'But if the Gods have discussed this question, whose explanation could be as good as yours? You are a great teacher. You can give me no greater gift than this understanding.'

Death was disturbed, and he counter-offered, 'I will give you sons and grandsons, all healthy and able to live a good and long life. You can have cattle and elephants and gold, as much land as you want. You can have wealth or anything your heart desires. I will give you beautiful women to tend to all your desires. But please don't ask me what happens beyond death.'

Nachiketa was not put off. 'These pleasures you offer me don't last. They are as fleeting as life on earth. We can't be happy with wealth when we know that death is around the corner. How can I, having approached an immortal like you, rejoice in a long life for the sake of pleasure? Please answer me. Does a person live after death or not? I ask nothing more than the secret of this mystery.'

Part Two: The Two Paths

Death was still reluctant to answer, but seeing that Nachiketa was so insistent, he decided to tell him a parable. 'A person comes to a place where there are two paths ahead: one path is the joy of the essence of one's being, and the other is the path of worldly pleasures. Those that choose the spiritual path connect to their essence, their inner truth, and find eventual and perennial peace, while those pursuing immediate pleasures do not.

'If you are wise you understand that you have this choice. There is a path of wisdom and a path of ignorance. You, Nachiketa, have chosen the path of wisdom to follow the true goal of life. There are ignorant people who go through life wise only in self-esteem and proud of their learning. They believe that they are their body and when their body dies, they are gone. But they are deluded.

There are those who understand that there is an eternal Self in all of us, but very few have experienced the joy of knowing their Self in Self-realization. The truth of the Self can only come to those who understand that they are the Eternal Self. This cannot be understood by the intellect, but only through the spirit in deep meditation. I hope one day to find another pupil like you who is wise in seeking his Eternal Self.

Nachiketa replied, 'I know that material pleasures are impermanent and I cannot reach an eternal state through them. This is why I have renounced all my desires for earthly treasures, so I can win the eternal through your instruction.'

Death said, 'You have rejected all my offers to fulfil any desire to dominate the world, to gain the rewards that come from ritual, and to have a life without fear and in the greatest of fame; in your wisdom you have turned me down. When the wise person meditates on God, contemplates the mystery of things and the soundings of his own heart, reaching deeper and deeper inside himself, he rises above pleasure and sorrow. Those who know that they are neither body nor mind, but are the Eternal Self, find the essence of joy and live in joy. I can see that your gates of joy are wide open.'

Part Three: The Eternal Spirit

Nachiketa asked, 'Tell me what is beyond right and wrong, cause and effect, past and future.'

Death said, 'I will tell you the one word that signifies all self-sacrifice, the word all the scriptures express, and that all spiritual seekers aspire to, and that is OM. It means Eternal Spirit, the highest place you can go. Finding the ultimate place connected to this highest power is more than one can ever desire. The Eternal Spirit is never born and never dies. Before the Eternal Spirit, there was nothing, and this Spirit lives on eternally and immutably. When the body dies, the Self, which is Spirit, does not. If a killer thinks he can kill, or the person being killed thinks he can die, both are wrong. The Eternal Spirit does not kill nor is ever killed.

'The Eternal Spirit hides in the heart of everyone. In deep meditation, when all the senses are quiet and one is free from desire, one can find this Spirit. Those who can surrender all human feelings find their Eternal Spirit, and realize that it is without form and does not change, even in the midst of change. It is these wise people who can move beyond sorrow. The Eternal Spirit is not found through the intellect or through learning. The Spirit comes to the person it loves and takes that person's body for its own. It can only be found through meditation, through concentration of the mind, the stilling of the senses, and profound peace in the heart.

'No one knows in truth where the Eternal Spirit is. The power of the Spirit takes away priests and warriors, and even death itself is carried away.'

Death continued, 'In the secret cave of the heart, two are seated by life's fountain. The separate ego and the Eternal Self live side-by-side, like shade and light. The ego lives in darkness and the Self in light. The enlightened sages say that those who worship the sacred fire in the name of the Lord cross the bridge to the shore where there is no fear, and they connect with the supreme everlasting Spirit.

'Consider the Self as if it is the owner of a chariot, and the body as the chariot itself. Reason is the charioteer and the mind is the reins. The horses are the senses and selfish desires are the roads they travel. The sages say that when we confuse the Self with the body, mind and senses, we experience suffering and enjoy pleasure, but have no real joy. When someone lacks steadiness and is unable to control his mind, his senses are like wild horses. But the mind can be trained, like horses. Those with little control over their thoughts do not reach the pure state of immortality, wandering from death to death. But those who manage to still their mind and have a pure heart, like a good driver with well-trained horses, reach their journey's end without dying and are united with the Lord of Love.

'Beyond the senses are the objects of desire, beyond the objects of desire is the mind, beyond the mind is the intellect, beyond the intellect is our true nature and our true Self. Beyond the true Self is the Eternal Spirit of the universe. This is where the path ends. The light of the Eternal Spirit is invisible and hidden in everyone. It is seen only by those who keep their mind concentrated on love and thus develop a super-conscious manner of knowing. Meditation enables them to go deeper and deeper into consciousness, from the world of words to the world of thoughts and then beyond thoughts to the wisdom in the Self, able to find inner peace.

'So wake up and find a good teacher. The path is hard. But those that find the formless, deathless, supernatural, undecaying, beginningless, endless, soundless, odourless, tasteless, intangible, unchangeable reality are forever free from the jaws of Death.'

Death continued, 'We were given senses to look outward, so many of us only look to the world outside and don't look within ourselves. You can only find your true Self by looking inwards. The ignorant person runs after pleasure and gets caught up in my nets. The wise person, understanding that the Eternal Self cannot die, does not chase after worldly pleasures that are impermanent. When the wise understand that it is only through the Eternal Self that we see, taste, smell, feel, hear and enjoy, they meditate on this Self and go beyond all suffering. When we are present with our Self, we are beyond fear and this is our true nature. The Eternal Self lives not only in our hearts but also among the physical elements. It is a boundless power manifesting as life itself, entering every heart, living there among the elements – that is the Eternal Self.

'We can meditate on the fire within us, which is the Eternal Self. We can meditate on the source of the sun and of every power in the cosmos, which is the Eternal Self. It is here and there, and there and here. We are not separate from the physical elements; this is the state of unity to aspire to. This is how we live without fear. As pure water poured into pure water becomes the very same, so does the Self of the enlightened man or woman become one with the Eternal Self.

'The person who meditates on the Eternal Self grieves no more, but is free. The Eternal Self is the sun shining in the sky, the fire on the altar, the guest in the house, and the wind blowing in the sky. He is the fish in water, the plant growing in the earth, the river flowing down the mountain. All these are the Eternal Self.

'It is this Self that controls our breath, and when our body dies, the Self lives on. Our lives are not controlled by the breath that flows in and out, but by the Self.

'Now, Nachiketa, I will tell you about the Universal Spirit and what happens to the Eternal Self after death. The Self may go to the womb of a mother and thus obtain a new body. It may even go into trees or plants, according to its karma. There is a Spirit who is awake in our sleep and creates the wonder of dreams. This is the immortal Spirit, Brahman. All worlds rest on this Spirit and no one can go beyond it.

'In the same way that fire takes on new forms in all things that burn, the Self takes new forms in all things that live. This Spirit, Brahman the Immortal, is within us all and out-side of us all. It is everything. There is one ruler, the Spirit that is in all things and who transforms His own form into many. Only the wise who see Him in their Self attain ever-lasting joy and peace.'

Nachiketa asked, 'How can I know that blissful state? Is the eternal soul light or does it reflect light?'

Death replied, 'There is neither the sun, stars nor moonshine. All these are given light from the light of the Spirit, and everything in the world reflects this light.'

Part Four: The Sacred Teaching

The tree of eternity has its roots above and its branches in the earth below. It is the Eternal Spirit who in truth is called the Immortal. All the world relies on the Spirit and no one can go beyond it.

The whole universe comes from that Spirit and its life burns through the universe. Its power is in thunder, fire, rain the wind and even death. If we can find this God, this Eternal Spirit, before we die, we are free from bondage. If not, we are born again and die again into new worlds and new creations.

When your Self is pure and you look in the mirror, perhaps you will see the Eternal Spirit within you in the same way that you see light and shade.

When the wise person knows that the material senses come from the ego and not from the Self, she understands about life and death, and no longer grieves. Above the senses is the mind, above the mind is the intellect, and above that is the ego, and above the ego is the essence, your Self, and beyond this the Eternal Spirit. Realizing this omnipresent eternal Self, one is released from the cycle of birth and death.

This Eternal Self is formless, and can never be seen with the eyes. But it is revealed in your heart when the heart is purified through meditation and the stilling of the senses. When the five senses and the mind are still, and the ego itself rests in silence, then your spiritual journey begins. This calm steadiness of the senses is called yoga, the union of mind, body and spirit. When she can stay in the state of union, the yogi can do no wrong. But before this state is reached, the unity of yoga comes and goes.

You must have faith in the Eternal Self. When all worldly desires are surrendered, then you become immortal, because although you are still in your body, you are united to the Self within you. This is the sacred teaching.

The heart has 101 channels, and one of these leads from the base of the spine to the crown of the head. If you can follow this energy channel, you win the immortal condition of self-realization, and find the Eternal Self within you. The Self that dwells in your heart should be understood as a pure immortal light.

And so Nachiketa learned the wisdom taught by the God of Death. He learned the method of meditation and the whole teaching of the inner union, known as yoga. In this he rose above desire and death and found the Immortal Spirit. So those who follow the path of yoga will also find their higher Self and the Eternal Spirit.

Those that understand this timeless tale of Nachiketa, narrated by Death, are able to live in spiritual awareness and find peace and joy.

Katha Upanishad

The Sound of Silence

The sage Prajapati was asked by the Valakhilyas, 'Since the body is like a chariot without consciousness, who has the power to make it conscious? Who is the driver of the chariot?'

Prajapati answered, 'There is a Spirit who is found amongst the things of this world and yet is above the things of this world. He is pure being and exists in the peace of a void of vastness. He is beyond the life of the body and the mind, never born, never dying, everlasting. This is the Spirit whose power gives consciousness to the body and he is the chariot driver.'

Then the Valakhilyas said, 'But how does this pure being give consciousness to the unconscious body? How is he the driver of the chariot?'

Prajapati answered, 'In the same way as a sleeping person wakes, but doesn't know, while still sleeping, that he is going to wake, so a part of the invisible Spirit comes as a messenger to the body without the body being conscious of its arrival. A part of infinite consciousness becomes our own finite awareness with powers of discrimination, definition and false conceptions. He is in truth you and me, the source of creation and the universal in us all. The Spirit is consciousness and gives consciousness to the body: he is the driver of the chariot.

The poets say that this is the Self who wanders on this earth from body to body, free from the light and darkness which follow our actions. He is free because He is liberated from selfishness and is also invisible, incomprehensible, hidden in darkness. He seems to work and not to exist; but truthfully He does not work at all, but simply exists. He is in his own being pure, never changing, never moving, unpollutable; and in peace beyond desires He observes the drama of the universe.

'The human self rules the body, but the Immortal Self is pure like a drop of water on a lotus leaf. The human self is under the power of the three forces of nature – harmony, activity and inertia – and thus it falls into confusion. Because of this confusion the self cannot become conscious of the Spirit who dwells within and whose power gives us the power to act. The self is whirled along the rushing stream of muddy waters of the three forces of nature and becomes unsteady and wavering, filled with confusion and full of desires, lacking concentration and disturbed with pride. Whenever the mind has thoughts of "I" and "mine" it binds itself with its lower self as a bird caught with the net of a snare.

'When a wise person has withdrawn his mind from all external things, and when his Self of life has peacefully left all inner sensations, he is able to rest in peace, free from the movements of will and desire. Since the living being has come from the universal Self, let the Self surrender itself into a state of Turiya, the fourth state of consciousness. It is said: there is something beyond our mind that sits in silence within our mind. It is the supreme mystery beyond thought. Let one's mind and one's subtle body rest on that and on nothing else.

'We can find the Eternal Spirit of Brahman in two ways: through silence and through the sound of OM. From sound we go to silence and with OM we go to the end: the silence of the eternal. The end is immortality, union and peace. The sound of the Eternal Spirit is OM and at the end of OM there is silence, the silence of joy. It is the end of the journey, where there is no more fear or sorrow: stay motionless, never falling, everlasting, immortal. God the Eternal Spirit is sound and silence. His name is OM. Therefore we must contemplate in silence on Him. In the same way that fire without fuel finds peace in its resting place, when our thought become silent the soul finds peace in its own source.

'And when our mind's longing for truth finds its real peace, then all false feelings caused by our former deluded actions come to a halt. Samsara, the transmigration of life, takes place in one's own mind. We must keep our minds pure because what we think, we become: this is the mystery of Eternity.

'When our minds are quiet, we overcome good and evil and in the quietness of our soul, we are one: then we can feel the joy of Eternity.

'If we think as much about God as we think of the world,

we might attain liberation. Our minds are both pure and impure: impure when we are in a state of desire and pure when free from desire. When the mind is silent beyond weakness or non-concentration, it can enter into a world which is far beyond the mind: the highest end.

'We should keep our minds lodged in our hearts until we have reached the highest end. This is the wisest thing we can do because it liberates us. Everything else is only words. Words cannot describe the joy of the Self whose impurities are cleansed in deep contemplation – who is one with his own Spirit, Atman. We only know this joy when we feel it.

'Our minds are the source of bondage and also the source of liberation. When we are bound to worldly things we are not free.'

MAITRI UPANISHAD

Breath Is Life

The person who finds the Eternal Spirit of Brahman, which is truth, consciousness and infinite joy, hidden in the innermost part of our Self and in the highest heaven, is granted all the blessings of life.

From the Eternal Spirit came space, from space came air; from air came fire; from fire came water; from water came earth; from earth came living plants, from plants came food and seed; and from seed and food came living beings, man and woman.

All bodies are made from food which becomes food again for others after their death. Food is the most important of all things for the body; therefore it is the best medicine for all the body's ailments. If you look on food as the gift of the universe, you shall never lack life's physical comforts. All bodies feed on food and it feeds on all bodies. Our physical body is made of food and contains within it the subtle body made of breath; prana, life energy, is the head, vyana is the right arm, the force of apana is the left, space is the heart and the earth is its bottom.

Man and woman, beast and bird, all live by breath. Breath has therefore been called the true sign of life. Breath is Life. It is the vital force in everyone that determines how long we are to live. If you look at the breath as a gift of the universe, you shall live a long life. The body is made of living breath.

The person who knows the spiritual joy that minds cannot grasp nor tongues speak, fears nothing. The thinking self is the soul of the living self, and within that lives the knowing self. Within the knowing self is wisdom. The knowing self grows up side by side with the thinking self, and the thinking self grows up side by side with the living self. Faith, truth, righteousness and discrimination are all there, while meditation is in its heart.

Being wise means living a life of selfless service. Those who attain wisdom and steadfastly worship the Spirit are freed from sin and find that all their selfless desires are granted. The knowing self is the soul of the thinking self and contains the joyous self, bliss. There is joy, contentment, delight and bliss in its heart and Spirit is its foundation.

Those who deny God, deny themselves. Those who affirm God, affirm themselves. Only the wise realize the Eternal Self. The Lord of Love willed 'Let me be many' and in the depths of His meditation He created everything that exists. Meditating, He entered into everything. It is He who gives reality to all.

Joy comes from God. We could not live or breathe if the joy of the Eternal Spirit did not fill the universe. If a man creates a gulf between himself and God, this gulf will bring fear. But if a man finds the support of the invisible and ineffable, he is free from fear. We must find that unity, the unity of Life.

Those who realize the joy of the Eternal Spirit know what is right and what is wrong, and have no fear. For words and thoughts that are not correct do not reach the person who is unified with this Spirit.

TAITTIRIYA UPANISHAD

The Unity of Life

One day Brighu Varuni went to his father and asked him, 'Father, please explain the mystery of the Eternal Spirit, Brahman, to me.'

His father told him about the food of the earth, the breath of life, and about seeing, hearing, speaking and thinking. He said, 'Seek to understand where these come from, by whom they live, and to whom they return. This is Brahman, the Great Spirit.'

Bhrighu went off and meditated and found that food is Spirit. From food all things are born, by food of the earth they live, and they return to the earth.

Following this discovery, he went back again to his father and said, 'Father, please explain further the mystery of Brahman.' His father said, 'Seek it through meditation, for meditation is Brahman, the Spirit.'

Brighu meditated further and found that life is Spirit. From life are born all creatures, by life they grow, and to life they return.

Not satisfied with his knowledge, he went back to his father and asked to be taught more of Brahman. His father repeated his answer, 'Seek it through meditation because meditation is Spirit.'

Brighu meditated and found that mind is Spirit. From mind are born all creatures, by mind they grow, and to mind they return.

Not fully satisfied with his knowledge, he went back to his father asking for more teachings of Brahman, and was told to meditate.

Brighu meditated and found that wisdom is Spirit. From wisdom come all creatures, by wisdom they grow and to wisdom they return.

Still not satisfied with his knowledge, Brighu went to his father appealing for more teachings of Brahman. Again his father told him to meditate.

So Brighu meditated and found that joy is Spirit. From joy all creatures are born, by joy they grow and to joy they return.

This is what Brighu found in the depths of his heart through meditation. When we realize this Spirit in our hearts we stand firm, grow rich and receive the love of all.

Respect food, the body lives on food; body is life; life is body; they are food to one another. Do not waste food; water is food, light lives on water. Water is light; light is water; they are good for one another. Store food; earth is food; air lives on earth. Earth is air; air is earth; they are food for one another. When we know this we shine in the light of the Spirit.

Never turn anyone away from your door. Gather enough food and invite the stranger in to eat. When you feed the hungry, you serve the Lord from whom is born every living being. When you give with purity, you get purity in return. When you give with energy, you get energy in return. When you give with ignorance, you are repaid with ignorance.

When we understand this teaching, our words become pleasing to others, our breathing deepens, our arms are ready to serve the Lord, and our feet are ready to aid everyone in need.

Realizing this, we see the Lord of Love in everything that the universe contains. When we draw on the Lord's resources within us, we have security, wisdom and love in action. We can conquer every enemy within to be united with the Lord of Love.

The Self in man and the sun are one. Those that understand this can see through the world and go beyond the layers of being to realize the unity of life. When we understand that all life is one, we are at home everywhere and see ourselves in all beings. Then we can travel beyond the universe and the light of the sun becomes our light.

TAITTIRIYA UPANISHAD

The Self Is the All in All

Who is the Self that we meditate on? Is it the Self by which we see, hear, smell, taste and through which we speak? Is Self the mind by which we perceive, understand, know, remember, will, desire and love? These are but servants of the true Self who is pure awareness. This Self is everything in everything. People who realize this eternal Self, called Brahman, live in joy and go beyond death.

AITAREYA UPANISHAD

The Lotus in the Heart

In the centre of the castle of the Infinite Spirit, which is Brahman, found in our own body, there is a small shrine shaped like a lotus flower in which there is a small space. We need to find out who lives there and we should desire to know Him. Why is it so important?

Because this little space within our hearts is as great as the whole vast world outside. Heaven, earth, fire, wind, the sun, moon and stars; whatever is and whatever is not, everything is there, for the whole universe is in Him and He dwells in our hearts.

The Spirit that lives in that space does not grow old and die. No one can ever kill the Spirit that is everlasting. The love of the universe dwells in the real castle of the Spirit, which we call Brahman.

The Self, the Atman, desires only what is real, and thinks nothing but what is true. Just as the attendants of a king obey their master and are with him wherever he goes, so all love is truth and all thoughts of truth obey the Self. If we depart this world not having found our spirit and that love which is Truth, we do not realize liberation.

CHANDOGYA UPANISHAD

The Wisdom of the Sage

There is a Light that shines beyond all things on earth, beyond us all, beyond the heavens, beyond the highest, the very highest heavens. This is the radiant light that shines in the heart of man.

The whole universe comes from the Higher Spirit, Brahman, and will return to the Spirit. We are creatures of will and we are only what we most deeply desire. It is our will and our deepest desire in this life that shape the life to come. So in silence we must direct our deepest desires with prayers, faith and vision to the Spirit, Brahman, to realize our Self.

The Self that dwells in our hearts is the Self that can only be realized in the silence of understanding that we are but spirit, and that our minds and hearts must be truthful and pure, finding, beyond words, joy in the essence of our being.

The Self dwelling in our hearts is smaller than a grain of rice, smaller than a grain of barley, smaller than a grain of millet, smaller even than the kernel of a grain of millet. But it is greater than the earth, greater than the sky, greater than heaven. This Self who gives rise to all works, desire, odours, tastes and who embraces the whole universe, who is beyond words, who is pure joy and who is always in your heart is the Higher Spirit, Brahman. When my ego dies and finds its restful place, I will find him. We should consider that in the inner world Brahman is consciousness, and in the outer world, Brahman is space. These are the two meditations.

CHANDOGYA UPANISHAD

Realize the Lord of Love

The Lord of Love is one. She is the supreme Lord dwelling in the heart of every living creature, who moves us to seek Her in our own hearts. She is the light that shines forever. She is the inner Self of all, hidden like a little flame in our hearts. We can only find Her when our minds have been stilled. Through Her grace, we are able to shed all selfish desires and sorrow and become united with the Self. The sage Shvetashvatara said that to know this Self is to be immortal and infinite. When we realize Her we become immortal.

SHVETASHVATARA UPANISHAD

You Are That!

Uddalaka had a son called Shvetaketu. When he was twelve, his father said to him, 'It is time for you to find a spiritual teacher. Everyone in this family has studied the holy scriptures and the spiritual way.'

So Shvetaketu went to a teacher and studied the scriptures for twelve years. He returned home very proud of his intellectual knowledge. His father observed him and said,

'My boy, you seem to have a high opinion of yourself; you are proud of your learning. But did you ask your teacher for the spiritual knowledge that enables you to hear the unheard, think the unthought and know the unknown?'

'What is that knowledge, Father?' asked Svetaketu.

'Just as by knowing a lump of clay, everything that is made of clay can be known, since any differences are only words, and the essential reality is clay. In the same way by knowing a piece of gold, all that is made of gold can be known, since any differences are only words, and the reality is only gold.'

Uddalaka responded, 'My teachers must not have known this or they would have taught it to me. Father, please teach me this knowledge.'

'I will,' replied his father.

'In the beginning there was only Being. Some people claim that in the beginning there was nothing at all and that everything has come out of nothing. But how can this be true? How can that which is, come from that which is not? In the beginning there was only one Being, and that Being thought, "I want to be many so I will create." Out of this creation came the cosmos. There is nothing in the cosmos that doesn't come from that one Being. Of everything that exists, this Being is the innermost Self. He is the truth, the Self Supreme. And you, Shvetaketu, you – are that!'

Shvetaketu asked, 'Please teach me more about the Self, Father.'

'Let's start with sleep. What happens when we sleep? When a person is absorbed in dreamless sleep, he is one with the Self although he doesn't know it. We say he sleeps but we mean he sleeps in the Self.

'A tethered bird grows tired from flying in every direction, finding no rest anywhere, and settles down at last on the very same perch on which it is tied. In the same way the mind, tired of wandering around here and there settles down at last in the Self, its life and breath, to which it is bound. All creatures have their source in that Being; He is their home; He is their strength.

'When a man is dying, speech folds into mind, mind folds into life, life dissolves into light, and his light merges into that one Being. That Being is the seed, the truth, the Self, and you, Shvetaketu, you – are that!'

'Please tell me more, Father.'

'My son, bees make honey by gathering nectar from many flowers to make their honey, so no one drop of honey can say that it came exactly from one specific flower. You can't identify the juice of one particular flower in the honey. And so it is with creatures like us who merge in that Being, whether in sleep or in death.

'And as the rivers that flow from the east or the west merge in the sea and become one with it, forgetting that they were ever separate rivers, so all creatures lose their separateness when they merge into pure Being. Whatever creature it may be – tiger, lion, wolf, boar, mosquito, worm – it only becomes aware of a particular life when it is born into it or is awake.

'If you strike at the root of a tree, it bleeds but still lives. If you strike at the trunk, the sap oozes, but the tree lives on. The Self as life fills the tree and supports it; it flourishes in happiness gathering food through its roots. However, if life departs from one branch, that branch withers, and when life leaves the whole tree, the entire tree withers. Remember my son, your body dies, but your Self does not.'

Uddalaka told Shvetaketu to bring him a fruit from a nearby banyan tree and to break it open. Shvetataketu did and said, 'There are seeds inside, all very small.'

'Now break one of the seeds and tell me what you see.'

'Nothing, Father.'

Uddalaka said, 'My son, this great banyan tree has

grown from a seed so small that you cannot see it. Believe me, an invisible and subtle essence is the Spirit of the whole universe.

'Now, take this salt and put it in some water and bring it to me tomorrow morning.'

The next morning Shvetaketu looked for the salt but couldn't find it because it had dissolved. Uddalaka asked his son to taste the water. 'Salty,' he said, adding, 'the salt will always remain in the water.'

'That's right. The salt permeates the water, just like the Self. Even though we cannot see it, the Self is within all things and there is nothing that doesn't come from Him.

'This invisible and subtle essence is the Spirit of the whole universe. That is reality. That is truth. And you, Shvetaketu, you – are that!'

CHANDOGYA UPANISHAD

Meditate on the Infinite

Is there anything higher than thought? Meditation is in truth higher than thought. The earth, sky, heaven, water, mountains seem to rest in silent meditation. When you meditate on the great and infinite Spirit, you find the peace, calm and inner joy that life can give you.

When we speak the truth, we speak words of greatness, because we know the nature of truth and desire it.

When we know, we can speak the truth so we must know the nature of knowledge and desire it.

When a man thinks then he can know, so we must know the nature of thought and desire it.

When we have faith, we think, so we must know the nature of faith and desire it.

When there is progress, we see and have faith, so we must know the nature of progress and desire it.

Where there is creation, there is progress, so we must know the nature of creation.

When there is the Infinite there is joy, so we must know the nature of the Infinite and desire it.

Only in the Infinite do we find joy.

When we realize the indivisible unity of life we see nothing else, hear nothing else, know nothing else – that is the Infinite. The Infinite is immortal; the finite is mortal. In our world what we call great is when we have possessions: land, gold and material goods. But this is not greatness, because in our world one thing depends on another. Only the Infinite is totally independent.

When we can find love and pleasure, union and joy in our inner Self, our Atman, or Spirit, we become our own master. When we can control the senses and purify our minds we can have a constant awareness of the Self; and where there is constant awareness of the Self, joy ends our sorrows and freedom ends our bondage, and we can find true liberation.

CHANDOGYA UPANISHAD

The Truth of All Truths

Once Gargya, a learned but proud man, went to Ayatasatru, King of Benares, and offered to teach him about the Spirit, Brahman. The king was interested in acquiring this knowledge so that his people would consider him most elevated. So he said to the sage, 'I will give you a thousand gifts if you can teach me.'

So Gargya began his teaching, 'I worship as Spirit the God that is in the sun.'

'No,' said the king, 'that is a very limited view. I worship Him as the crowned king of all.'

Gargya continued, 'I worship as Spirit the God that is in the moon.'

'No, that's not the right way to talk about the Spirit,' responded the king. Gargya went on to suggest that the Spirit to worship is in lightning, wind, fire, water, mirror, shadow and finally life and the power of intelligence. But the king dismissed all of these as inadequate, so Gargya, exhausted by his efforts, asked the king to teach him instead.

The king took him by the hand to go for a walk, and they soon came upon a man who was sleeping soundly. The king called him by different names, but the man didn't stir until they shook him awake. The king said, 'You see, when the man was sleeping his consciousness had gone, but when we woke him it returned. Where does this consciousness go and where does it come back from?' Gargya didn't know.

The king said, 'When he was asleep, he moved around in his dreams. His world was a dream world. Using his senses, he wandered around in the world of dreams. But once he entered into a deeper sleep he became conscious of nothing at all. His soul rested peacefully in his heart and he entered into the Self. All the powers of life are really truth and their truth is the Spirit or Self. If a man worships the Eternal Spirit thinking that the Eternal Spirit can be one thing or another, he does not realize the truth, nor can he reach the bliss of liberation.

'In the same way that threads emerge from a spider, and sparks shoot from fire, so all the senses come from this Self. He is known as the truth of all truths. The senses are true but he is the truth of them all.'

BRIHADARANYAKA UPANISHAD

The Supreme Magician

May the Lord of Love from whom all things come and into whom they all return, grant us the grace of pure vision.

He is fire, sun, moon and stars. He is the air and the sea;

He is this boy, that girl, this man, that woman, this old man – His face is everywhere. He is the blue bird, the green bird, the thundercloud, the seasons and the seas. He has no beginning and no end.

He is the Creator, the source from which the worlds evolve, and His face is everywhere. The magic of name and form, of you and me, casting the spell of pain and pleasure, all come from Maya, his Divine power. It is only when we are able to see through this magic veil that we can see the One who appears as many.

There are two beautiful birds, two good friends, living in the very same tree. One eats the fruits from the tree, while the other looks on in silence. The first represents the human ego who, actively pursuing pleasure, feels sad with her lack of wisdom. The other, the Lord of Love, stays silent and when we see her in all her majesty, we are able to free ourselves from sorrow.

All scriptures are useless if we do not experience the Spirit from which we all come, have been, and will be. With Maya, the goddess of illusion, His uncanny power of wonder, He made all things, and by Maya the human soul is bound. We must understand that nature is illusion, but the Eternal Spirit is the ruler of Maya, and all beings in the universe are parts of His infinite splendour.

We must know Him to be the supreme magician who has brought forth from His uncanny power boy and girl, bird and beast. He bestows all our blessings and His grace fills our hearts with profound peace. May this God of all gods grant us the grace of pure vision.

Who is this God that we must adore? It is He who rules this world of man, woman and all living beings. He is the God of infinite forms, smaller than the smallest atom and the Creator of all. In the vision of this God of Love is everlasting peace. He is the guardian of the cosmos. When we realize Him we cut the bonds of death and are free from all bondage. He is far beyond the reach of the mind. He alone is. His glory fills the world. He is far beyond the reach of our eyes. May He reveal Himself to us in the depths of our meditation and grant us immortality.

SHVETASHVATARA UPANISHAD

The Immortality Lesson

Yajnavalkya said to his wife Maitreyi, 'Dear, the time has come for me to depart this worldly life and retire to one of meditation. I want to divide my worldly possessions between you and our family.'

Maitreyi said, 'If I received all the wealth in the world, would it help me to become immortal?'

Yajnavalkya replied, 'Not at all. You would live and die like any other rich person. Money does not buy immortality.'

Maitreyi said, 'Then material possessions and money are not useful to me. Will you teach me the ways that leads to immortality?'

Yajnavalkya answered, 'I have always loved you, but now I am overjoyed to hear you ask this question. Come sit with me and reflect deeply on what I am going to tell you.'

'A wife loves her husband, but it is not for the love of her husband that her husband is dear, but for the Spirit that is in the husband. It is the same for children, wives, wealth, religion, power, animals, and everything else. Nothing is loved for its own sake – it is only the Self, or Spirit, that is loved. When this Self or Spirit is seen and heard in our thoughts and meditation, then we know and understand everything that exists.

'When we hear music playing, we do not identify the individual notes separately from the tune. Only in the whole are the parts known. The Self or Spirit is that whole. Only by knowing the Self can all the separate elements be known.

When we live in a state of individuality, we can see and hear and feel and know another. But when we realize that everything is Spirit, and that Spirit is identical with one's own Self, then how can we see, hear, feel and know another?

'When a lump of salt is thrown into water, it dissolves and cannot be removed even though we can taste the salty water. So the separate Self dissolves in the sea of pure consciousness, infinite and immortal. Separateness comes when we identify the Self with the body; when this physical identification dissolves, the Self is no longer separate.'

BRIHADARANYAKA UPANISHAD

Rebirth

The true nature of the Self is to be free from fear, free from desire and free from evil. As lovers in deep embrace forget everything and only feel peace all around, when a person embraces his true Self he feels peace all around. In that state of peace there is neither father nor mother, and there are no gods. He can neither see, hear, taste, smell, know or feel. Yet he can see – for sight and he are one; he can hear – because sound and he are one; he can taste – for taste and he are one; he can smell – for smell and he are one; he knows – for he and knowledge are one; he can touch – for he and touch are one.

The Self is eternal and immortal, man's highest goal and deepest bliss. Most creatures can only experience a small part of this bliss, so human beings are very lucky indeed.

When a person is about to die, the lower self groans like a heavily laden cart. Then the Higher Self takes charge and prepares for the final journey. The dying person becomes weak and seemingly unconscious. His powers and senses unite with his subtle body. Then by the light of the Self, life departs from the body. But the Self remains conscious and with consciousness the dying man goes on his journey. The deeds of his life and their results go with him.

Just as a caterpillar when it reaches the end of a blade of grass moves on to another blade and moves his body from the first, so the Self, having reached the end of this body, enters a new one. Or as a goldsmith takes an old vase, melts it down and reshapes it into a new one, so the Self after death eventually comes back in a new vessel, perhaps a human body, perhaps a celestial being.

We act according to our desires. After death we go to the next world bearing the subtle impressions of our prior deeds. We return with the same desires, and thus continue birth after birth. However, when we have conquered desire, we do not return and are allowed to become one with the Higher Spirit. The path from desire to liberation is long and hard. It is only by treading this path that we can realize the Higher Spirit. Those who tread this path have no desire for children, wealth or power; evil is burned away and we are freed from desire, sorrow and doubt.

BRIHADARANYAKA UPANISHAD

Rebirth and Immortality

Two things are hidden in the mystery of infinity of the Eternal Spirit: knowledge and ignorance. Ignorance passes away and knowledge is immortal, but the Eternal Spirit in eternity is above both ignorance and knowledge. He is the One who presides over all and rules over everyone from inside; He sows the golden seed of life when time begins, and helps us to know its unity. The Lord of Love fills the hearts of all created beings just as the sun shines everywhere, filling all space with light.

When we live selfish lives as if hypnotized by pleasure and pain, we are not free. Although we appear the masters of ourselves, we go from birth to birth driven by our own deeds and karma. The Self, though a very small flame in our hearts, is like the sun shining brilliantly. When it becomes one with the ego, the self-conscious 'I am' and its desires, the Self appears other than what it is. It may be smaller than a hair's breadth but it is infinite.

The Self is not male or female, but it takes the form of a body with desires, attachments and delusions. The Self is born again and again in new bodies to work out the karma of past lives. The quality of the soul determines whether its future body will be earthly or airy, heavy or light. Its thoughts and actions can lead it to freedom or lead it to bondage, life after life. Love the Lord and become free. He is an incorporeal Spirit but can be seen by a heart that is pure. He is God, the God of love, and when a person knows Him he leaves behind his past life bodies and becomes immortal.

SHVETASHVATARA UPANISHAD

The Godly and the Godless

The great teacher Prajapati said, 'The Self is pure, free from decay and death, free from hunger and thirst and free from sorrow. This is the Spirit in man. The only thing this Spirit desires is truth. This is the Spirit that we must seek and know: we must each find our own Self. When we have found our Self and got to know it, we have reached the ultimate, and there is nothing more to desire.'

The godly and the godless both heard what Prajapati said and thought, 'We must find that Self, that Spirit, so that we can obtain all our desires.'

So Indra, the godly, and Virochana, the godless, both went independently to Prajapati, carrying gifts as a sign that they wanted to be his pupils, and for thirty-two years they lived as religious students with him. At the end of the thirty-two years, Prajapati asked why they had stayed with him for so long.

Indra and Virochana answered, 'We have heard your inspiring words: the Self is pure and beyond old age and death, free from hunger, thirst and sorrow; a Spirit who desires only truth, and whose thoughts are truth. You say that we must find this Spirit and understand it because when we do all our desires will be met. This is why we have become your pupils.'

Prajapati said to them, 'When you look into another person's eyes what you see is the Self, fearless and deathless. That is the Higher Spirit, Brahman, the Supreme.'

They asked, 'What is it that we see reflected in a mirror?'

'It is the Self that you see in all of these. That same Self is seen in all. Go and look at yourselves in a bowl of water and tell me what you see.'

They did, and responded, 'We see ourselves clearly, our doubles, even our hair and our nails.'

'Then dress up, put on beautiful clothes and jewellery, and look at yourselves again and tell me what you see this time.'

They did, and answered, 'We see ourselves as we are, all dressed up.'

'That is also the Self, fearless and deathless.'

Indra and Virochana went away satisfied, but Prajapati said to himself, 'They have seen the Self, but they have not understood. They have not yet found their Spirit. They mistake the Self as the body. If you think that the Self is the body then you lose your way in life.'

Virochana, certain that the Self is the body, went back to the godless and began to teach them that the body alone is to be saved and adored. He taught them that if you live with indulgence of the senses you will find joy in this world and the next. Even today, when we lack faith, love and charity, we are called godless.

Before Indra returned to the godly, he could see the danger of this teaching and thought, 'If our Self is the body and it is dressed in beautiful clothes, then when the body is blind, the Self must also be blind, and when the body is lame, then the Self must be lame, and when the body dies, our Self dies also. I don't understand the spiritual benefits of this teaching.' So he went back to Prajapati with gifts in hand as a sign that he wanted to be his pupil again.

'Why have you come back?' asked Prajapati. 'You left here satisfied.'

Indra replied, 'Lord, if the body is all adorned, so is its reflection; but if the body is blind, lame or crippled, the Self would be blind, lame and crippled; if the body is dead, the Self would be dead. I don't see any benefits to this understanding.'

'You are correct. Stay with me for a further thirty-two years and I will teach you more about the Self.' So Indra lived with Prajapati for a further thirty-two years, and after this time Prajapati said to him, 'The Self is that which moves about in joy in the dreaming state, fearless and deathless.'

Indra went away satisfied, but later began to question this knowledge and went back a third time to Prajapati. 'Why have you returned? Aren't you satisfied?' the sage asked Indra.

Indra replied, 'In the dreaming state, the Self is not blind when the body is blind, nor lame when the body is lame; yet in this state the Self may seem to be killed and suffer and even weep. I can find no joy in this teaching.'

Then Prajapati said to him, 'Live with me for a further thirty-two years and I will teach you more about the Self.' So Indra lived with him for another thirty-two years, and at the end of this time his teacher said, 'When a person is fast asleep, at peace with himself, serene and dreamless, that is the Self, the Immortal beyond fear. That is the Eternal Spirit, called Brahman.'

Now Indra left with peace in his heart, thinking he was ready to start teaching about the Self, but before he reached his pupils, he saw the danger of this teaching and he returned once more to Prajapati. Again Prajapati asked why he had returned and Indra replied, 'When you are in a state of deep dreamless sleep, you are not aware of yourself or of anyone else. I think that in this state you are very close to extinction. I don't see any knowledge in this teaching either.'

'You are thinking very clearly, Indra,' said Prajapati. 'Live with me for a further five years and I will teach you to realize the Self.' So Indra lived with Prajapati for another five years, making a total of 101 years that he lived with his teacher. People often said that the Great Indra lived with Prajapati the pure life of a spiritual student for 101 years in order to learn to master the Self.

After this time Prajapati revealed the highest truth of the Self to Indra: 'It is true that the body will die, but within the body lives the imperishable Self. The body experiences pleasure and pain, so no one that is ruled by his body can ever be free from pleasure and pain. But those that know they are not the body can pass beyond pleasure and pain to live in a state of joy.

'The wind, clouds, thunder and lightning have no body, but when they rise up and reach the light, they show their own shapes. Likewise when the Self is in silent quietness it arises, leaves the body and, reaching the Spirit Supreme, it finds its body of light. This is the land of infinite liberty where, beyond the mortal body, the Spirit of man is free. There he can laugh and sing and forget that while he was on earth, he was attached to his body. As a beast is attached to a cart, so on earth the Self is attached to a body.

'When we see, smell, speak, hear or think, it is the Self that sees, smells, speaks, hears and thinks. The senses are only the instruments of the Self. It is because of the light of the Spirit that the human mind can see and think and enjoy this world. When you know your own Self in truth and light, you experience peace and joy.'

CHANDOGYA UPANISHAD

What the Thunder Said

The children of the Creator – gods, humans and the godless – all lived with Him as students.

When the gods had completed their studies, they said, 'Venerable One, please teach us.'

The Creator answered with one syllable: **DA!**

'Do you understand?'

'Yes,' they said, 'you have told us to be self-controlled.'

'You have understood,' He said.

Next the human beings said, 'Venerable One, please teach us.'

The Creator answered again: **DA!**

'Do you understand?'

'Yes, you have told us to give.'

'You have understood.'

Then the godless approached. 'Venerable One, please teach us.'

The Creator said the same syllable: **DA!**

'Do you understand?'

'Yes, you have told us to be compassionate.'

'You have understood.'

The heavenly voice of thunder repeats this teaching:

DA!! DA!! DA!!
Be Self-controlled!
Give!
Be Compassionate!

OM Shanti Shanti Shanti
Let peace and peace and peace be everywhere.

BRIHADARANYAKA UPANISHAD

A Prayer

O Lord of Love who is revealed in all the scriptures, who has assumed the form of all creatures, grant me the wisdom to choose the path that will lead me to immortality.

Make my body strong, my tongue sweet, my ears sharp. May my ears always hear the sound of OM, the supreme symbol of the Lord of Love, and may my love for Him grow more and more.

May I grow in spiritual wisdom. May I never lack clothes, cows, food and drink so that I may serve you better. May students come to me from far and near like a flowing river all the year. Help me to guide them to live in peace, control their minds and senses that they may be able to serve you better.

Oh Lord of Love, may I enter You and may You reveal yourself to me. In Your waters may I wash my sins away. Take me and enlighten me.

TAITTIRIYA UPANISHAD

II

The *Bhagavad Gita* (the *Celestial Song*)

The action of the *Bhagavad Gita* takes place sometime between 1000 and 700 BCE, and its setting is Kurukshetra, the field of the Kurus, not far from present-day New Delhi. The *Bhagavad Gita* forms part of the epic *Mahabharata*, traditionally ascribed to the sage and seer Vyasa.

1. The Conflict of Arjuna

Two vast armies, the Pandavas and the Kauravas, were lined up facing each other, about to engage in battle. Insults and battle-cries were hurled across the field, and there was a cacophony of sound as conch shells roared, cow horns bellowed, cymbals clashed, trumpets blasted and drums pounded. Huge numbers of horse-drawn chariots, archers and foot soldiers were drawn together in close formation, in readiness for the charge, while flags and banners waved in the wind.

Prince Arjuna and his brothers, the heads of the Pandava clan, prepared for battle. Arjuna stood in a chariot pulled by two snow-white horses, the reins held by his driver, Krishna. He and his brothers all blew their conch shells, which roared like lions. Arjuna took up his bow and arrows, in readiness for battle, and said to Krishna, 'Krishna, drive my chariot into the middle of the field, where I can see my enemies face to face.'

Krishna jerked the reins and the horses pulled the chariot into the field. Nearing the mid-point, Krishna pulled the horses up and said, 'Arjuna, look at the entire Kuru family assembled here in one place.'

Arjuna looked over at the opposing side, and saw his own kinsmen lined up against him: grandfathers, uncles, teachers, in-laws and friends. Overcome with compassion and sorrow, he said, 'Looking at my own people here eager to fight, I have a sense of dread. My limbs have lost their power, my body trembles, my mouth is dry, and my hair stands on end. My mind is reeling, and I can hardly stand.

'I don't see what good can come from killing my own relations in war. Oh Krishna, I don't desire victory, or to gain a kingdom or pleasures. Why should I want a kingdom, or pleasures, or even life itself, if the very people I would want them for – teachers, fathers, sons, grandfathers, uncles, in-laws, grandsons and others – are battling against me and putting all their resources against me? Even if they were to kill me, I would not want to kill them, not even to rule over all the worlds.

'O Krishna, what delight can I find in killing my relatives? I would become a sinner by slaying these men, even though they are evil.

'These people are family; therefore, I should not kill them. Killing my own family members can only make me miserable.

'Although they are overcome by greed and see no evil in destroying our family or by injuring their friends, I recognize the horror of it. Why shouldn't I turn away from this?

'We seem determined to kill our own relations out of greed for the pleasure of ruling a kingdom. I think it would be far better if the Kauravas were to kill *me* in battle.'

Arjuna, overwhelmed with despair and grief, threw down his bow and arrows, and sank down on the floor of the chariot.

2. Yoga of Wisdom

When Krishna saw his friend Arjuna so despondent, his heart so overcome with sadness and grief, and with tears filling his eyes, he said to him, 'Where has this feeling of hopelessness come from, and at such a dangerous time? Don't give in to weakness, it doesn't suit you. You're a man. Throw off these discouraging feelings and stand up.'

Arjuna looked up and replied, 'How can I attack my great uncle and my teacher? It would be better for me to live as a beggar than to kill these great men who have been my teachers. Even if I did kill them, the rest of my life would be stained with their blood. I don't know which is better – for us to slay them or for them to slay us. My first cousins and the king are all here. Would I want to live after I have killed them? In the darkness of my soul, I feel empty. In my self-pity I don't know the way of righteousness. Krishna, I am your disciple, please show me the right path! Even if I were to become rich and have no rival here on earth or in heaven, I can't see an end to the overwhelming grief that fills my soul.'

After unburdening his heart to Krishna, the Lord of the senses, Arjuna declared that he would not fight, and fell silent.

Krishna smiled and spoke to Arjuna. 'You grieve for those who have no need for grief. Are your words really wise? The wise don't grieve for the dead or the living – for life and death pass away. There was never a time when I did not exist, nor you, nor any of these ruling princes. Nor will there ever be a time in the future when all of us cease to exist. After the Spirit of our mortal body moves through childhood, youth and old age, the Spirit wanders on to a new body: the wise do not doubt this. Sensations come and go: they are impermanent. Our senses give us a feeling of heat and cold, pleasure and pain. Patiently endure them and rise above them, Arjuna. The person who can remain balanced and still when he feels pain and pleasure is able to experience immortality. When we see the truth, we know what is real and what is not. The Spirit is indestructible. No one can destroy what is everlasting and imperishable. The Eternal Spirit lives in the bodies of these warriors, and although their bodies will die, the Spirit remains immortal. So, great warrior, you must carry on the fight.

'It is not correct to think that you can kill or be killed. For the Eternal Spirit in man cannot kill and cannot die. The Eternal is never born and can never die, and the Spirit is not killed when the body is killed. When we truly know the Self, the Eternal Spirit that is indestructible, eternal and changeless, how then can we kill or be killed? Who would be killed? In the same way that we discard old clothes and dress in new ones, the Spirit leaves the mortal body and enters into a new one. Weapons and fire cannot hurt the Spirit. It is untouched by water and wind. This Spirit can't be pierced or cut; it can't be burned, moistened or dried. The Spirit is everlasting, omnipresent, immovable, ever One. The Spirit is said to be imperceptible, unthinkable and unchanging. Therefore when we know it is like this, there is nothing to grieve for.

'Even if you imagine that the Atman, the Self, is born and dies, there is still no reason to grieve. Whatever is born will die, and whatever is dead will be reborn. You should not mourn the inevitable. All beings are invisible before they are born and again after they are dead. They are only visible when they are in the midst of life, so what is the point of sorrow? We may see the Self as full of wonders, while others may speak of it as marvellous. Yet none completely understand it. This Self, which lives in each one of us, is eternal and indestructible, Arjuna. Therefore you do not have to grieve for anyone.

'You must also think of your duty and not falter. There is no greater good for a warrior than to fight in a righteous war. There is a war that opens the gates of heaven, and the warriors whose fate it is to fight such a war are happy warriors. But if you don't fight when it is your duty to do so, you will lose your honour and integrity and bring disorder to your life. People will always tell the story of your dishonour, and for an honourable man like you, dishonour is worse than death.

'If you are seen to withdraw from battle through fear, those that have held you in high esteem will think much less of you. Your enemies will scorn your strength and slander you. What could be more painful for a warrior than a shameful fate? In death you will find glory in heaven, while in victory you will find glory on earth. So rise up, Arjuna, and be ready to fight.

'Prepare for war with peace in your soul. Remain at peace in both pleasure and pain, and in victory or in loss. In this peace there is no sin. You have been given the wisdom of yoga: listen to it, act on it, and you can break through the constraints of karma. Following the path of yoga, no effort made is lost and there are no adverse effects. Even a little practice of this dharma preserves one from fear. If your mind is chattering all the time and unsteady, there are too many choices and thoughts. But when your mind is clear and one-pointed, there is only one way to go.

'There are men who follow the scriptures and speak as though there is nothing else and no other way. With their minds full of desires and heavenly treasures, they speak mostly of rites and rituals, believing these will bring them pleasure and power. Those people who are attached to pleasure and power cannot sit in meditation with their minds concentrated, and enjoy the peace that brings. Rise above the forces of Nature and be centred in your own eternal truth, and you will be balanced, free of wanting to get or keep anything. Because when you are already enlightened, the scriptures are as irrelevant as a well in a flood.

'Do your work, but don't go looking for any benefits from the results. Don't be motivated by the fruits of your actions, but you must never become inactive either. Do your work in the peace of yoga, free from selfish desires, not moved by success or failure. Yoga is evenness of the mind, a peace that is always steady. Work done for reward is greatly inferior to work done through the yoga of wisdom. Take refuge in wisdom, because those who are motivated by the rewards of their work are to be pitied. With this wisdom and stillness of mind, we can go beyond good and evil. So practise yoga, for yoga is perfection in action.

'Those who act with wisdom in union with the Divine, not worrying about these rewards, become free from the bonds of birth, and reach the state where there is no sorrow. When you are enlightened enough to transcend delusion you become indifferent to whatever you have heard of, or will hear of in future. When your mind becomes still and centred, and is no longer confused by the conflicting information in the scriptures, then you experience yoga.'

Arjuna was intrigued, and he asked, 'Can you describe the person who is steady in wisdom and who maintains the state of samadhi? How does someone like that speak, sit or walk?'

Krishna responded, 'A person who has been able to let go of all personal desires, and is completely content in the truth of his Self, is someone whose soul has found peace. A person whose mind is not troubled by sorrows and has no longing for pleasure and happiness, who is beyond passion, fear and anger – that is someone of steady wisdom. One who is free of all mental attachments and neither rejoices when good things happen, nor feels despondent when bad happens, maintains a serene wisdom. The person who can withdraw his senses from the world of pleasurable sensations, like a tortoise drawing its limbs within its shell, has unwavering wisdom. When we stop feeding on these pleasurable sensations, they drop away, although the longing for them doesn't. But even that longing disappears when our soul connects with its highest truth. Even for the wise, if their senses become excited, their minds get carried away too.

'The yogi learns to control the senses by meditating on Me as the highest goal. As her senses are controlled, her wisdom again becomes steady. When a person dwells on the pleasures of the senses, she develops an attachment to them; this attachment leads to desire, and desire results in anger. Anger gives rise to confusion, and confusion to loss of memory. When we lose our memory, we lose our powers of reasoning, and when reason is gone, we are absolutely lost.

'But the yogi who has disciplined the mind and has gained control of her senses is no longer tossed back and forth by pleasure and pain, and can settle deeply in serenity. In that serenity, her sorrows disappear; she has found tranquillity, wisdom, and peace in her heart.

'You cannot find wisdom or meditate if the senses are out of control. Without this contemplation there cannot be peace, and without peace there is no joy. The mind that follows the wandering senses loses all reason, like a ship that is tossed about on rough seas.

'Therefore, one who has gained control of her senses is steady in her wisdom. To the enlightened person, what seems like night to others is the state of awakening, and what appears as day to others is as night to those who know the Self.

'We cannot experience true peace when we have desires. But when all desires merge like rivers flowing into the ocean, we are ever one in infinite peace. We can all experience peace if we live without personal desires, free of 'mine-ness' and egoism.

'This, Arjuna, is the ultimate state. When you experience it, you will have no further questions. Even in your last hour of life on earth, with this awareness, there is just the merging into the oneness of God.'

3. Karma Yoga – the Yoga of Action

Arjuna asked, 'If you tell me that the path of wisdom is better than the path of action, how can you encourage me to go to war? This is confusing, as it seems to be contradictory. Please tell me truthfully what path I need to take to become blissful?'

Krishna answered, 'In this world there are two paths: the path of knowledge – Jnana Yoga – and the path of selfless action – Karma Yoga. We cannot become free by inaction, nor can we become perfect by rejecting action. No one can live without action, since we are all driven to action by the impulses unleashed by the forces of nature.

'If you still your body when seated in meditation, but your mind continues to think about external objects, you are deluding yourself and are not really following the path. But great is the person who is free from attachments, who controls his senses and engages his body in Karma Yoga, the action of selfless service. Do your duty – this is better than doing nothing, since your body cannot live without action. Work that is not performed in the spirit of sacrifice puts the world in bondage. Therefore let your actions be pure, and free from worldly desires.

'The Lord of Creation made humankind through His own sacrifice, and said that through sacrifice you can grow and obtain your desires. With sacrifice you will honour the Gods, who will then honour you. When you work in harmony, and love them with all your heart, you will reach the highest goal. Happy with your sacrifice, the Gods will love you, and in harmony with them you will attain the supreme good. Remember that anyone who receives from the Gods without giving anything back is a thief. The good people, who eat what remains after the sacrifice, are freed from past sins. But the sinful, who cook food for themselves alone, create more sin.

'We are born of food; food is produced from rain; rain is the result of selfless sacrifice; and sacrifice is the result of actions. Know that the origin of karma comes from Brahman, imperishable and eternal. Therefore Brahman, Spirit, is always the primary focus of sacrifice.

'If we fail to align ourselves with the wheel of life, which is reflected in the ever-revolving cycle of sacrifice leading to action, action leading to God, and God once again leading to sacrifice, but instead choose to waste our lives as slaves to our senses, we are worthless. When we have found the joy of the Spirit and are satisfied with this, having found peace, we are beyond karma. Similarly, we have nothing to gain here on earth either by doing or not doing, nor do we depend on anyone for anything. So do your duty without attachment. If you do things without expectation of results you will reach the highest state.

'King Janaka and others found enlightenment through Karma Yoga, the path of selfless action. Let your aim in life be the good of all and carry out this work. People follow whatever a great person does, and they use his standards as their own. Consider my case. I have no duty left to perform on earth, or on the astral or celestial planes. I have nothing to obtain because I have it all, but I still work. If I stopped doing my work, everyone would follow that example and stop theirs too. And if my work came to an end, these worlds would end in destruction, and confusion would reign; this would be the death of all beings.

'The unenlightened do things with attachment to results. The enlightened, however, do things with the same energy but without attachment, and so guide others on the path of selfless action. The wise person does not disturb the mind of the unwise while they perform their selfish work. Instead, working with devotion, he shows them the joy of doing good work.

'The forces of Nature accomplish everything. But when our minds are clouded with ego, we think that we have made things happen. Arjuna, the person who understands the relationship between the forces of Nature and actions, and sees how the forces of Nature work together with other forces of Nature to make things happen, does not become their slave. If we are deluded about these forces of Nature then we become attached to Nature's functions. But when we understand how Nature works, we should not disturb the mind of someone who doesn't have this awareness.

'Surrender all your actions to Me, and, with your mind fixed on the Self, free from desires and the idea of ownership, you can engage in battle. When you live by these teachings, with faith and goodwill you can find freedom through pure work. Those who do not follow My doctrine and criticize it misunderstand everything. They are confused in mind and are lost. Even the wisest act according to their own nature. All beings follow their own nature. Why try to force things to be otherwise?

'The senses are always attracted or repulsed by various external objects. But don't let them dominate you or they will become your enemy. Following your own path, imperfect though it may be, is better than following someone else's, however great theirs may be. It's better to die in one's own duty: to live in another's is death.'

Arjuna asked, 'What power is it, Krishna, that drives a person to act sinfully, even against his will, as if he were powerless?'

Krishna replied, 'It is greedy desire, and anger born of passion, the great evil: this is the enemy of the soul. Just as fire is covered by smoke, a mirror by dust, and an embryo is surrounded by a membrane, so human wisdom is covered by the insatiable fire of desire, the constant enemy of the wise. The senses, the mind and the intellect are the seat of desire. It is this desire that clouds our wisdom and deludes us.

'So, Arjuna, take control of your desires, the destroyer of vision and wisdom. The power of the senses is great, but the power of the mind is stronger, and stronger still is the intellect, but the Self is superior to them all. So knowing that the Self, Atman, is beyond reason, let His peace bring you peace.

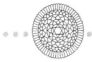

Be a warrior and kill your desires, the powerful enemy of the soul.'

4. Wisdom Yoga of Action and Renunciation

Krishna continued, 'I taught this yoga science to Vivasvan who passed it to his son Manu, the father of man. And Manu taught his son, King Ikshvaku, the saint. Yoga science was passed from teacher to disciple over the years, until even the saintly kings knew it. But over time the succession was broken, and this doctrine was lost. However, I am giving you this wonderful secret of yoga because you are my devotee and I am your friend.'

Arjuna was confused. 'But you were born after Vivasvan, so how is it possible for you to have taught this to him?'

Krishna replied, 'I have lived many lives, as you have too. I remember mine, whereas you don't. The truth is that I am eternal, unborn and everlasting: I am the Lord of everything. I appear in this earthly form through maya, my own power of illusion. When righteousness is lost and evil prevails, I manifest on earth in bodily form; I come into being from age to age to protect the good, destroy the wicked and establish righteousness. Those that truly know Me are not reborn after death, but come directly to Me. Many people have come to Me, trusting in Me, filled with My Spirit, free from passion, fear and anger, purified by the fire of wisdom. I, as God, am the peace within us. In whatever way people worship Me, they find My love: for many are the paths but in the end they all lead to Me.

'Those who desire success offer sacrifices to the Gods, and success soon follows from their efforts. I distribute the qualities and activities of the forces of nature throughout humanity. Be aware that I created the forces of Nature but I do not control them. I am free from the bond of work because I have no expectation of the results. The person that sees this truth finds freedom in his work. Even those of ancient times who understood this freedom continued to work in the world. Like those sages, you should work too.

'Even the wise are confused as to what constitutes action and inaction. I shall explain karma to you so that you will be free from evil. One needs to know what is meant by action, and to discern the wrong kind of action, as well as what is meant by inaction. Karma is a mysterious path. The person who in movement finds rest, and who understands that movement grows from stillness and rest, sees the light, and finds peace in all his actions. The sages say that whoever does things without personal desire for success is wise. That person's actions are pure and he knows the truth. In whatever work he does, such a person has peace: he expects nothing, and he relies on nothing. He does nothing, although he is always engaged in action. Having given up desire, with control over his mind and ego, he is free from all attachments, and only his body works. He is free from sin. He is happy with whatever the universe has given him and is not attached to pleasure or pain; he is happy whether he succeeds or not, and is not bound by his actions.

'When you let go of all attachments and experience liberation, you find peace in wisdom. Then everything you do is a sacrifice and all your karma disappears. The person who sees God in all his work goes truthfully to God: God is his worship, his offering, offered by God in the fire of God. Some yogis make sacrifices to the Gods, but others offer their very selves as sacrifice to the Eternal Spirit. Some restrain their senses, whilst others sacrifice worldly objects that would otherwise be enjoyed by the senses. Wisely, some restrain their senses or their vital energy as a sacrifice. Others offer their wealth as a sacrifice, or their suffering, or the fruits of their yoga practice, or the knowledge of sacred study. For those interested in the regulation of the breath, pranayama, they offer the incoming breath to the outgoing breath and the out-breath to the in-breath. Breath sacrifices itself to support our life: the breath enters our body and we burn it up.

'Others who limit their food intake sacrifice their energy through self-control. All these yogis are purified by self-surrender. If you do not make some sacrifice, neither this world, nor the next, will be beneficial to you. Those who enjoy what remains of the sacrifice go into the Eternal Spirit. People sacrifice themselves in many different ways, according to their karma. Knowing that all sacrifice is holy work, you shall be free.

'It is better to give knowledge than to give wealth or material goods, because all sacrificial actions lead to wisdom. If you want the wise to teach you the path to enlightenment, bow to them with humility, question them and serve them. This is the only way to receive their teachings of sacred knowledge.

'When you realize this truth, Arjuna, you will no longer be confused. You will see all things in your heart and your heart in Me. With this wisdom, even if you have been the worst sinner in the world, you will sail past all sin and evil. Just as a burning fire reduces its fuel to ashes, the fire of eternal wisdom burns all your karma to ash. There is nothing as purifying on this earth as wisdom. The person who lives in self-harmony finds this truth in his soul.

'Anyone who has faith and is able to control his senses finds this wisdom, which leads to the realization of deep peace. Through ignorance, there are those who have no sincere belief, and live with constant doubts; they are lost. There is no joy for those who live with doubts, not in this world, not in the future. If all your actions are appropriately dedicated to Me, then your work becomes karma yoga. In this way all doubts are destroyed through your wisdom and awakening; you are no longer tied by the constraints of the mind and you become realized in the true Self.

With the sword of wisdom, kill all the doubts that are born of ignorance in your heart. Be one in self-harmony, in yoga, and stand up, great warrior!'

5. Yoga of Renunciation

Arjuna said, 'You recommend both the path of renunciation and the path of unselfish action. Tell me, which one is better?'

Krishna answered, 'Both lead to freedom. Of the two, Karma Yoga, selfless action, is better. A true renunciate has no cravings and does not hate anyone or anything. In this way he has freedom. The wise say that renunciation and Karma Yoga are the same. If you follow either path with all your soul, you will receive the fruits of both. The yogis who follow the path of renunciation and those that follow the path of Karma Yoga reach the same heightened states of consciousness: they see both paths as one and the same. But renunciation is difficult to attain without Karma Yoga, the performance of selfless actions that purify the mind. The sage who meditates regularly with a purified mind soon realizes God.

'Through the practice of karma yoga and meditation, the mind becomes pure and well-disciplined, the senses become quiet, and you can see that your Self is one with the Universal Self.

'The person that is in harmony with his inner Self believes that he does not do any work, for in seeing, hearing, smelling, touching, eating, walking, sleeping, breathing, talking, holding on, letting go, and even in opening or closing his eyes, he knows that it is his body and mind that is working, not his true Self. The person who lets go of attachment to success or failure, and instead dedicates his actions to God, is not touched by sin, just as the lotus leaf is not touched by water.

'The yogi works only for the purification of her Spirit without attachment to results, so it is only her body, her senses, her mind or her reason that works. The person disciplined in yoga becomes totally at peace by renouncing desire for the rewards of her work. One who is not yet disciplined desires rewards for her actions, and has no inner peace.

'By controlling her senses and renouncing the fruits of her actions, the yogi's mind becomes disciplined, and she can rest in the joy of silence in the castle of her body; she does not do selfish work nor cause another to do it.

'It is the work of Nature that creates the forces that are active in the world, and not the work of the Supreme Spirit. The Lord does not measure good and evil in people. Their wisdom is darkened by their ignorance, and this is what leads people astray. Those whose ignorance is made pure by the wisdom of their inner Spirit, know who they are and become enlightened. Their wisdom is like the sun and in its radiance they see the Supreme.

'Those whose thoughts are on the Self, finding their inner purpose with It and becoming one with It, are no longer subject to rebirth, and their sins are washed away by true knowledge. When you have realized the Self, you see the Self equally in a priest or a cow, a dog, or even in a man who eats dogs. When you understand that we are all unified with the Eternal Spirit everywhere, you become equitable towards all because you are unified with all, and can rise above the constant changes of this world.

'When you become established in the Absolute, your reason is steady and there is no delusion. Those who have found this state are unattached to pleasure, and do not suffer pain. When we are no longer attached to external things, we find an inner peace and joy. Pleasure that comes from worldly things brings us sorrow because they come and they go, being transient; the wise man finds no joy in pleasure. Whilst on this earth, if you can endure the storms of desire and anger, you are a true yogi, a joyous soul. The yogi who has this inner happiness and joy has found his inner light. Such a yogi has become godlike, and attains the release that comes from being at one with the Eternal Spirit. Those who have realized their unity with the Eternal Spirit are really wise; their sins have been washed away, their soul is in harmony, and their joy is in the good of all.

'When your mind is calm and controlled, free from desire and anger, you can easily realize your true Self, and enjoy the bliss of being at one with the Eternal Spirit. When you withdraw your attention from external things and put your focus on the third eye that lies between the eyebrows, and balance the ebb and flow of the breath, you can control the mind, the senses, and the intellect. Then, with desire and anger gone, your soul is silent, and you experience the final liberation.

'Those who know Me as the Lord of Self-sacrifice, as the Master of the Universe and the friend of all, reach a state of total peace.'

6. Yoga of Meditation

Krishna continued, 'The person who works without expecting an earthly reward, but does the work that needs to be done, is a Sannyasi, a renunciate, a true yogi. Those who live without sacrifice or devotion are not true yogis. Renunciation is the discipline of yoga; no one can become a yogi without renouncing his personal desires and will.

'Karma Yoga, selfless service, is the path the wise follow to attain the state of yoga; reaching that state brings deep peace. You reach the true state of yoga when you are no longer bound by the senses, or by your earthly work, and when you have completely surrendered your earthly will.

'Your mind can behave as a good friend, but also as your enemy. As you gain control of your mind with the help of your higher Self, you are a friend of your higher Self, and your mind and ego become your friends. The uncontrolled mind acts as your enemy. When your mind is disciplined and your soul is at peace, you are peaceful, and remain unaffected by heat or cold, pleasure or pain, praise or blame. A true yogi is completely happy with the wisdom of spiritual knowledge and has developed total control and calm over his senses; to him, gold, stones or earth are one and the same thing. He views relatives, companions and friends, those who hate him, and those who are impartial, with the same sense of inner peace.

'A serious yoga practitioner must continue to concentrate her mind on yoga in deep solitude until she becomes the master of her mind and body, hoping for nothing, desiring nothing. When you practise meditation, set up a clean place with the seat neither too high nor low, and place some insulation on the spot between the body and the ground, so that the meditation area becomes charged with meditative vibrations.

'Sit on this spot calming your mind and senses by concentrating on one point: this is the practice of yoga meditation to purify your spirit. While meditating, sit up straight with your head and neck relaxed and still, poised at the top of your body, with your gaze softly focused on the tip of your nose. Sit this way in yoga meditation, serene and fearless, with your mind calm and your thoughts fixed on Me – the Divine. Through steady and continuous practice, the mind will stop wandering and will find a peaceful state. This practice will naturally lead you to nirvana, the peace supreme that is in Me.

'Yoga is a harmonious practice. It is not for the person

who eats too much or too little, or who sleeps too little or too much. When we are moderate in food and play, disciplined in our actions, sleep enough but not too much, and avoid extremes in everything we do, we will find that yoga practice takes away all our pain and suffering.

'When the mind of the yogi is in harmony and finds rest in her inner spirit, without wanting for anything, then she is established in yoga and unified with God. The yogi who practises yoga of the Self has a still and controlled mind, unwavering like the steady flame of a candle in a windless place. When the mind is still and quiet, the Spirit reveals itself in joy and peace. Then the yogi finds, in the depths of her heart, the infinite joy that is above and beyond the senses, and she never strays from her innermost truth. Wanting for nothing, unshaken by any situation, life itself becomes a meditation.

'Freed from the oppression of pain, you find yoga in its true sense, the union with God. This must be consistently practised with faith and a strong and courageous heart. Letting go of all desires that arise from our thoughts, and controlling the senses with the mind, we are able to become tranquil and still, focusing on the Self without thinking of anything else. And when chattering thoughts come to distract us, we bring the attention back to the Self again.

'So for the yogi whose heart is still and at peace, she experiences the greatest joy and becomes one with Brahman, Infinite Consciousness. Directing her mind this way, the yogi's sins disappear and she happily experiences the infinite bliss of union with Brahman. Then she sees herself in the heart of all beings and sees all beings in her heart; she sees the same Self everywhere and in everything.

'Those who see Me in everything and everything in Me, know that the Self in each individual is the Self in all things, and they never again feel separate from Me, or Me from them. Through understanding the oneness of love, the unity of all created beings, and by worshipping Me abiding in all living things, the yogi lives in Me. Knowing they are one with Brahman, the yogis understand oneness with the universe and as such experience the pleasures and pains felt by others as if it were their own. This is the highest spiritual union.'

Arjuna asked, 'But the mind is so restless and constantly changing, how is it possible really to still the mind and keep it stilled? Often it is more than restless, it is turbulent and very obstinate. Controlling it seems as impossibly difficult as trying to tame the wind.'

Krishna answered, 'The mind is restless and very hard to train. With constant and dedicated practice, non-attachment and firm faith, it can be done. It is difficult, but it is possible. For those who cannot master their ego and control their mind, the Self-realization of yoga is extremely difficult. But if you persist with your practice and with non-attachment, the wayward mind will become still, and you will reach the state of understanding the Self that is Yoga.'

Arjuna asked, 'What happens to the yogi who with great intent and sincere belief is still unable to quieten his mind, or who dies before reaching perfection through yoga? Will this yogi have failed in both this world and future worlds? Does he perish like the cloud that is dissolved by the wind, not having found the path of God? Be the light in my darkness and destroy my doubts, please, Krishna.'

Krishna replied, 'Have no fears, Arjuna my friend, for the one who has embarked on the path of yoga will not come to a bad end in this world, or any world beyond. For all those who embark on the path of yoga, and die before reaching the highest state, reach the heavenly state of the virtuous and stay there for some years. Then they will be reborn into a home that is pure and prosperous, to continue their quest. Or they may be reborn into a family of wise yogis, although this is a rare occurrence. But they will begin their new lives with the wisdom of their former lives and will continue to strive for spiritual perfection. The yoga practitioner is carried forward by the strength of his earlier practices. Those who show interest in yoga and spiritual matters advance further spiritually than those who follow only rites and ceremonies, without thought or understanding.

'So with persistent effort over many lifetimes, a yogi will become purified of all desires, and achieve the ultimate goal of becoming one with the Eternal Spirit. Be a yogi, Arjuna, for the yogi is superior to the ascetics, and to the men and women of knowledge or action. And the greatest yogi of all is he who with all his soul worships Me with complete faith and becomes one with Me.

7. Yoga of Knowledge and Realization

Krishna said, 'It may seem impossible to you but everyone can come to know God. How? Listen to Me, focus your mind on Me, take refuge in Me, and practise yoga. Then you will undoubtedly unite with Me, and come to know Me fully and completely. I will teach you the wisdom and knowledge that will lead you to the supreme truth. Once you combine and understand both of these in your daily life, there is nothing more that you need to know in this world.

'Perhaps only one in a thousand will seek to reach perfection, and probably only one out of a thousand who reach it will gain true knowledge of Me. First, you must learn that I have two aspects: a higher Self and a lower self. The lower self is made up of eight basic components of Nature: earth, water, fire, air, space, the mind, intellect and the ego. But beyond my visible and material nature is My more subtle and higher Self, and this is My invisible Spirit that gives life to the entire universe.

'All things have their life in this life and I am their beginning and their end. Apart from Me, there is nothing whatsoever. I hold the entire universe in the same way as a string holds the gems of a necklace. I am the innate nature of everything. I am the taste of pure water; the radiance of the sun and the moon; I am OM, the sacred word; I am the sound of it heard throughout the universe; I am the courage in the centre of all people. I am the pure scent that comes from the earth, the brightness of the fire and the sun; I am the life in all living beings, and the purifying force in the austere life of those who train their souls.

'So, Arjuna, know me as the everlasting seed of eternal life; I am the intelligence of the intelligent and the splendour in all that is beautiful. I am the power of the strong, free from personal desire and attachment. I am also the desire in all beings, when that desire is set on doing good for the universe. And the three forces of Nature, the three states of the spirit, come from Me: fine, serene light; restless, passionate activity; and dull, inert darkness. These qualities of nature come out of Me, they are My manifestations. But I am not within them: I do not rely on Nature in any way: it relies on Me.

'Most people do not realize that if they look beyond the ever-changing qualities of Nature, they will find Me, the transcendent one: I am never changing. The veil of illusion is hard to see through. Only those who in truth surrender to Me are able to see through it. Others, who are deluded by illusion, lose their ability to discriminate, sink to their lower nature, and commit evil deeds. They don't seek refuge in Me or have any faith.

'There are four reasons why people worship Me: to overcome suffering, to understand life, to seek worldly objectives like wealth and power, and, for those already wise, to become even more spiritual. The greatest of these are the wise, because they know My truth and are devoted to Me. I am as dear to them as they are to Me.

'All sincere seekers of spirituality have good and noble

souls; but those who know the truth, and with a steady mind know Me as the essence within themselves, are always with Me, are the closest to Me, and seek Me as the highest goal. After many lives, a person becomes wiser and takes refuge in Me and nothing else. They see that all the world is their innermost Self. These people are rare.

'Others, whose personal desires still lead them astray from good judgement, worship lesser gods for their blessings. If a person desires to worship with great faith this or that God, I will make their faith steady and unwavering. Imbued with that faith, he worships the Gods he has chosen and obtains the fruits that he desires, but whatever is good comes from Me. But these are people of little wisdom and the good they want has an end providing only fleeting satisfaction. Those who worship the gods, go to them; My devotees come to Me. The unwise have not yet understood that My existence is supreme and unchanging, and so they only think of Me as a worldly body. Not everyone can see Me as I truly am, because I cover myself with a veil of illusion, so most people do not recognize Me as the one who was never born, and never changes. I know all that was, is, and is to come, but no one knows Me.

'All beings are born with the sense that the world around them is 'real', thereby losing their connection with the Divine. Our likes and dislikes become desires and we come away from the absolute truth: that we already have peace and happiness in our spirit, but our ego has got in the way.

'But when we dedicate our actions to the Divine, we rise above the delusion of our own habits and desires. Those who are scared of old age and death, and come to Me, learn of their True Self: Atman, and the Divine Brahman and karma.

'The yogis know Me in earth and in heaven, and in the fire of sacrifice. They have no fear of death, because they know that as their bodies fall away, their consciousness becomes one with My cosmic consciousness, and they are liberated from rebirth.'

8. *Yoga of the Absolute Truth*

Arjuna asked Krishna, 'Who is Brahman? Who is the Self: Atman? What is the essential nature of karma? What is the Kingdom of the earth? And what is the Kingdom of Light? What is the essence of Self-sacrifice? How do we make such an offering? And how are those who control their minds during death able to unite with you, my Lord?'

Krishna responded, 'So many questions, Arjuna! Brahman is My absolute highest nature, the supreme, the eternal, vaster than vast, omnipresent, imperishable, inde- structible, eternal, Divine. The essence of each created being is the Atman, the Self, which is the Brahman inside each and every one of us. Karma is the first action that starts everything off. Through my initial creation, which is the first karmic act, all beings are created and the entire universe is established. The perishable earthly realm is the physical body, but Spirit is the Kingdom of light. I sacrificed My body to create this universe and I am the essence of Self-sacrifice present in your body.

'Your last question about death is very important, so know this: if you think about Me at the very moment of death you will leave your body and come to Me, and will experience peace and tranquillity. A person is united with whatever he is thinking about at his time of death. Whatever occupies your attention throughout your life will inevitably be your consciousness at the moment of death, and to that realm of consciousness you will go. So think of Me constantly and fight for what is right. Have total faith in Me, be deter- mined to achieve a quiet mind and a pure and truthful heart, and then you will come to Me in death.

'If you are disciplined and practise steadying your mind, without allowing it to wander to fruitless thoughts, you go to that Spirit of Light. The person who meditates on the One who is all-perceiving, the ruler of all things, smaller than the atom, whose form is beyond darkness and shines like the sun; the one who, at the time of his death, is in a union of Love with the power of yoga, and with a steady mind keeps the power of his breath focused on his third eye, that person is merged in the radiant Supreme Being.

'Now I will tell you about the reality known by those who understand the essence of the holy scriptures. The eternal truth can be experienced by those who learn how to control their minds, live in peace from earthly passions, and strive for perfection. At the time of death you should close down the gates of your senses, put your mind into your heart, and from there direct the energy and breath to your head. Then chant the sacred word OM, which is the manifestation of Brahman, and you will leave the body and achieve the supreme goal.

'This is really the essence of My teachings. If you constantly and steadfastly remember Me, at every moment of your life, you will merge with Me with ease. Those who come to Me, the Abode of great joy, are great souls, and are so perfected that they never return again to this world of human sorrow. Every being on earth returns to nothing, even the world of Brahma, the creator God. But after they have merged with Me, there is no rebirth.

'Those who know that the day of Brahma, the God of Creation, lasts a thousand ages, and that his night also lasts a thousand ages, truly know what day and night are. When this day comes, all creatures are manifested out of the invisible; and when the night of darkness comes, all again merge into the invisible. So the beings who live again and again, all merge into oneness at the approach of each night, and then return again as separate forms at the dawn of another day.

'But beyond birth and rebirth there is yet another unmanifested eternal reality that continues forever and does not vanish, even when all things pass away. This is the everlasting and highest Supreme goal which is My very nature. The one who has realized this has come home, never again to be separate, never to return again. You can have this experience through an eternal love in the Spirit Supreme. In Him all things have their life, and from Him all things have come.

'There are two paths for the individual Self at the point of death: freedom from reincarnation or bondage. The yogi who is on the path of light and truth, when leaving his body, goes directly to Brahman. Selfish and ignorant souls go into darkness when they die, and are chained to the cycle of birth and death. These two paths of light and dark are eternal in this world. One leads to liberation, and the other to rebirth. When you know these paths you will never again be deluded. If you persevere in your practice of yoga, Arjuna, you will gain this great knowledge.

'There are many benefits that come from studying scriptures, performing selfless service, performing deep cleansing and purifying practices, and being charitable. But through the practice of yoga, and understanding the paths of darkness and light, you reach the greatest state of all, coming home to the Divine love that lives in your heart.'

9. Yoga of Royal Knowledge and the King of Secrets

Krishna told Arjuna, 'As your Spirit has faith, I will tell you the most profound and mysterious secret. This knowledge will free you from the sorrows of the world and from wrong-doing. This is the highest form of knowledge that you can learn from the experience of your dharma, your own inner truth, which is easy to follow, and leads to the

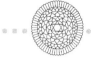

highest end. Those who have no faith in this Truth do not find Me; they are compelled to return to the cycle of death and rebirth.

'The visible universe comes from My invisible Being. All beings in the worlds exist, in spirit, within Me, and depend on Me. I am the source of all beings, I support them all, but I do not rest in them. Just as the mighty wind rests in space, so all beings have their rest in Me. Know this truth.

'At the end of the night of Brahma, the God of Creation, all things return to My Nature, and when the new day dawns, I bring them back into the light of life. Over and over again I give Nature the power to bring life to all creation, infusing Spirit into everything and subjecting all creation to the laws of their own nature. I am not bound by this huge work of creation, since I exist with no attachment to My actions.

'I watch as Nature creates everything that moves or is still; and because of this, the world keeps revolving. But the fools of the world don't look beyond physical appearance, so they overlook my true Nature, which is the Lord of everything. Being deluded with the self-preoccupation of their ego, their lives are fraught with pain. Their minds are never calm and peaceful, living a life of ignorance, only seeking to satisfy their worldly desires. Their works and hopes are all in vain.

'But the great souls are led by their Divine Nature, and knowing My true Nature, they worship Me with one-pointed devotion. They praise Me with devotion and their vows are strong. Always engrossed in yoga, their harmony is ever one, and they worship Me with all their love. Other great souls on the path of wisdom worship Me with the sacrifice of their spiritual vision. They worship Me as One and as many; wherever they look they see My face.

'I am the sacrifice and the offering, the sacred gift, the food that is medicinal and nourishing; I am the sacred chants; I am also the pure offering into the fire, the fire into which it is offered, and the one who receives it.

'I am the father of this universe and even its most ancient grandfather; I am the mother and Creator of all. I am the one who gives you the results of your actions, your karma. I am the only thing that is really worth knowing and the only thing to know, since everything else is part of me. All humanity is purified by contact with Me. I am the sound of OM, and I am the most sacred of scriptures.

'I am the goal at the end of the path; I am the Master, your only lasting refuge: all beings dwell in Me. I am the best friend who lives in your heart, the beginning, middle, and end of all things; I am their seed of eternity and their supreme treasure. I cause the heat of the sun, and send and hold back the rain. I am immortality and death; I am being and non-being, what is and what is not.

'Those who follow rituals, offer worship, and pray for heaven in time reach celestial planes and enjoy the pleasures of heaven. But when the rewards of their work come to an end, they return to this world in the cycle of rebirth and death, caught by their attachment to the pleasures of heaven. I look after the well-being and security of those who adore Me, and who meditate on Me with the pure oneness of their soul, always immersed in yoga.

'Even those who worship other gods with a pure and loving heart worship Me, because I am the object of all worship, and the one who accepts every sacrifice: I am their Lord supreme. But because they do not know my pure Being, they fall back into the cycle of rebirth.

'Those who worship the deities go to the deities. Those who worship their ancestors are reunited with them after death. Those who worship the spirits go to the spirits. But my devotees come to me, the Supreme Reality.

'I joyfully accept whatever is offered to me with true devotion, whether it is a leaf, a flower, or a sip of water, because it is given in love. So whatever you do, Arjuna, whatever you eat, sacrifice, give up or give away, even your suffering, give it devotedly to Me. This is the way to be free from the bonds of karma and its good and bad results. Finding release through the yoga that has no expectation of the results of your actions, and letting go of your desires, you will come to Me and merge with Me.

'I am the same towards all creatures. I neither dislike nor favour any of them. But those who worship Me with devotion realize that they are actually part of Me, and that I live in them. Even if the worst sinner devotes his life to Me with a pure heart, he becomes transformed into a saint, and before long becomes a person of righteousness and discovers lasting peace. I promise you that one who loves Me shall not perish.

'It does not matter about your birth, race, sex, caste, or whether you are sinful, weak or humble – if you come to Me with true faith, you will attain the Supreme Goal. Even the holy men through their devotion seek the very same goal. So finding your Self in this world of change and suffering, just turn yourself to Me, and take joy in Me. Think of Me constantly, devote your life to Me, offer all your actions to Me, surrender to Me. Performing your yoga in this way you will become steady on your path to the Supreme goal, and enter into my very Being.

10. Yoga of the Divine Manifestations

Krishna said to Arjuna, 'Keep listening, great warrior! As you seem delighted by my teachings, I will elaborate further. Neither the gods nor the holy men know My origin because in truth I am the source of them all. Those who understand that I am without birth or origin, the great Ishvara and Supreme Lord of all the worlds, are free from delusion and evil. All these different qualities of man come solely from Me: reason, wisdom, freedom from confusion, forgiveness, truth, self-restraint, control of the ego, happiness, unhappiness, birth and death, fear and fearlessness, non-violence, tranquillity, contentment, simple austerity, generosity, honour and dishonour.

'Understanding this mystical information, you can see My Divine power: whatever you sense or perceive in this world is that same power: and so you have yoga, the union with the Divine. I am the source of everything: I am Love. Yogis who give their minds and hearts fully to the Divine know that God is the source of everything. With their attention and life energy flowing into Me, absorbed in Me, these yogis always speak of Me with joy, and their lives are filled with peace and contentment. To those who are sincerely devoted and worship Me simply out of love, I give the yoga of vision, and with this they come to Me.

'With compassion I chose to dwell in your heart, and from there I remove the darkness of ignorance with the great light of wisdom.'

Arjuna said, 'You are the Supreme Brahman, Light Supreme, and Supreme Purifier, Spirit Divine Eternal; You are beginning-less and Your presence is everywhere. All the sages say this about You, and You Yourself also say it to me. O Krishna, I know that everything You tell me is the truth. Neither the most powerful demons nor the gods themselves can fully grasp the truth of You. You and only You know who and what you are, Master of the Universe, source of all beings, ruler of all.

'Please tell me more about the divine forms in which You live and through which you pervade all that is. How should I meditate to know You? Which of your forms should I put my attention on? Tell me again of Your power and Your glory, for I never tire of hearing of them. Your words are the nectar of my life.'

'Krishna answered, 'I shall describe to you the most significant of my Divine manifestations, for there is no end to them. I am the Spirit that dwells in the heart of all things. I am the beginning, the middle and the end of all that lives. Above man's senses I am the mind, and I am the light of consciousness in all living creatures. I am Vishnu, the all-encompassing light, the radiating sun among the bright gods of light, the bright moon in the lights of the night. I am the whirlwind, the Lord of the winds, who brings good to the world.

'I am the God of destruction, dispelling evil from the mind; I am the Lord of wealth. I am the fire of the radiant spirits bringing warmth and life. I am the highest of the high mountains.

'I am the Divine priest, the Lord of devotion. I am the God of war, leading the world to victory over the demons. Of all the bodies of water, I am the vast ocean into which all the rest merge.

'Of all the great sages, I am the teacher of yoga. I am the sound of OM, the word of eternity. Of all sacrificial offerings, I am the recitation of mantras, the prayer of silence. And of things that do not move, I am the Himalayas, the highest.

'Of trees, I am the tree of life. I am the principal teacher of unity. I am the King of the celestial beings. I am the best of the best. Among men I am the king of men.

'I am God's thunderbolt coming down on wickedness. Among creators, I am the Creator of Love; and among serpents, the serpent of eternity.

'I am the God of water. I am the noble ancestor. And of the governing forces of the universe, I am the Lord of death. I am the Prince of devotion. Of all that measures I am time itself; the lion, the king of the beasts; of birds I am the Lord's eagle. Among things of purification, I am the wind, and among warriors I am Rama, the supreme hero who only uses his weapon for the good of humanity. I am the shark, the most powerful of the sea creatures, and of the rivers I am the sacred Ganges.

'I am the beginning, middle and end of all that is created; I am the knowledge of the Self that makes ignorance disappear. And I am reason itself. I am the first letter A; I am the combining word: *and*. I am time eternal, the Giver who faces all directions. And I am death that will take everyone, yet I am also the source of all that is yet to be born; I am the feminine qualities of fame and fortune, eloquence and memory, intelligence, perseverance and forgiveness.

'I am the best of the *Vedas*, the most sacred of all poems. I am the best month for spiritual practice, and of the seasons, I am the spring, when the new flowers bloom.

'I am the roll of the gambler's dice. I am the splendour in all that is splendid. I am determination and victory. I am the goodness of those who are good.

'I am the sceptre, the symbol of measured justice amidst those who punish others. I am the secret of silence and the wisdom of the wise.

'So know, Arjuna, that I am the seed of all things that are, and that no one and nothing that is movable or immovable, can ever be without Me.

'There is no end to my manifestations. Know that all things beautiful and good, prospering or powerful, are only a small portion of My radiance.

'But Arjuna, what is the point of knowing all these details? Just know that I am and that I stand and support the whole of this universe with a sole fragment of Myself.'

11. *Yoga Vision of the Cosmic Form*

Arjuna said, 'In your great compassion You have taught me the deepest mystery of the Self, which has removed my delusion. Having heard at length of the origin and passing away of all creatures, and of Your infinite greatness, it now makes sense to me, O wondrous lotus- eyed Lord. Now that I see that everything is as You said it is, my soul is longing to see You in Your true form of God, rather than this Krishna body. Lord of all yogis, if You think I am strong enough to see it, then please show me.'

Krishna replied, 'You will see the hundreds and thousands of my forms, of various Divine kinds, endless colours and variations. You will see within Me all the celestial powers and spirits of Nature and so many other wondrous things that have never been seen before. Look at My body: you will see the whole universe there, all that moves and all that is unmoving, as well as anything else you desire to see.

'But you cannot see My cosmic form with human eyes. I need to give you special spiritual vision, my divine yoga.'

And so Krishna, the God of Yoga, appeared to Arjuna in his supreme Divine form. And Arjuna saw in that form so many visions of wonder: everywhere eyes from innumerable faces seeing everything, countless mouths all speaking wonders, numerous celestial ornaments, and more visions than can be described.

Krishna held several weapons up high, symbolizing His infinite powers. He was dressed in mantles of light, adorned with garlands of flowers of heavenly fragrance, and He faced in every direction simultaneously. The light shining from the Supreme Spirit was like a thousand suns blazing in the sky. And Arjuna saw in the radiance of Krishna's cosmic body the whole universe in all its variety and myriad forms.

Arjuna, overwhelmed and amazed, bowed his head and put his hands in a prayer position at his heart and spoke, 'O Lord, I see in Your body all the Gods, every living creature, and even the Creator, Brahma, sitting on the lotus and surrounded by the ancient sages and celestial serpents. All around I see Your Infinity: I see You embodied in so many forms. You are everywhere: bodies, arms, mouths, eyes and the fire of life of Your innumerable bodies. There is no beginning, middle or end of You, O God of all, Lord of the Cosmos.

'I can see You crowned with precious gems and holding the mace and discus. Your radiance is glowing so brilliantly I can hardly look. You are like a fire, a blinding sun blazing out in all directions. You are the imperishable, the Supreme among what can be known, the support of this vast universe, the Eternal guardian of timeless wisdom. You are the everlasting ruler of the law of righteousness, the Spirit who is and who was at the beginning. I see You as without beginning, middle or end, with inexhaustible power, innumerable arms, the moon and sun for Your eyes, Your mouth a blazing fire heating up this world.

'Heaven and Earth and all the spaces in between are filled with the vast limitless presence of Your Spirit; and the three worlds tremble before Your terrifying and wonderful form. All the Gods, angels, and higher beings enter into You, joining their palms in joy and wonder, praising You. Hosts of sages and saints come to You, singing Your praises with hymns and glorifying You. Even the myriad of celestial beings gaze at You with awe and wonder.

'The whole universe is trembling, Lord, on seeing Your immense form and infinite strength with its many eyes, mouths, arms, thighs, feet, bellies, frightening teeth: I also tremble. When I see Your vast form taller than the sky, burning with so many colours, with wide-open mouths, huge flaming eyes burning into me like fire, my heart shakes in terror and I lose my courage and peace. When I look into Your mouths with all those sharp teeth resembling the destructive flames of Time, I wonder where I am. Where is my shelter? Have mercy on me, God of Gods, Supreme Refuge of the World.

'All of my enemies, and all the earth's warriors and kings, are helplessly caught up in Your jaws; some are caught and their heads crushed into powder. Like a raging torrent roaring to the ocean, so these heroes of our world rush into Your flaming mouths. Now I can see that all creatures are rushing to Your fire in their own destruction, just as moths rush towards the light. You swallow up people on every side, licking at them with Your blazing mouths. Your heat pervades the whole universe, setting it on fire with Your radiance.

'O God, who are You in this form of terror? I adore You, O God Supreme: I want to know You, the Fundamental Spirit, for I do not understand what You do and why You do it.'

Krishna said, 'I am all-powerful Time, which destroys all things, and I have come here to destroy this world. Even if you do not fight, all these warriors on the opposite army will die. So get up, win your glory, conquer your enemies, and enjoy your kingdom. They are already doomed to die because of their karma: I have already killed them. You are to be My instrument, Arjuna. So go ahead and slay the brave warriors that I have already doomed to die in this battle. Don't be afraid. Just stand and fight and you will conquer your enemies in battle.'

When Arjuna heard these words, he pressed his palms together over his heart, bowed down before the Lord, and, with a trembling voice, said: 'It is right, O God, that people shower praises on You. All evil spirits fly away in fear; but the hosts and sages bow down before You. How could they do anything else but bow down and worship You? You are beyond everything else. You are the origin of all things, even creator of Brahma, the God of infinite Creation. You are home to the universe, God of Gods, being without end; You are all that is and all that is not.

'You are the first of the Gods, the Fundamental Being, the Supreme Haven of the universe. You are awareness itself – the knower and all that is known. You are the infinite Presence in whom all things are.

'God of the winds and the waters, of fire and death; Lord

of the moon, the Creator, the Ancestor of all; I salute You a thousand times, and again and again I respectfully bow to You. I prostrate in front of You, behind You, and on every side. All-powerful God of immeasurable strength: Your prowess is beyond measure. You permeate all that is. In truth You are everything. If sometimes in the past I addressed You as "Krishna, son of Yadu, my friend", I did it out of ignorance and carelessness but with affection, not realizing who You really were. I am sure that my manner at times was too familiar when we were resting or playing, sitting or eating. In whatever way I have been disrespectful to You, Lord, please forgive me.

'You are the father of the world and all that is in it, movable and unmovable. There is no one who is Your equal in the three spheres. How can there be anything greater than You? I bow down before You and beg for Your forgiveness, as a parent forgives their child, as a friend forgives his friend, or a lover forgives a beloved.

'I am so happy to have been given the chance to see what no one has ever seen before – Your cosmic form; and yet I am filled with fear. Please show me Your more familiar form again, O dear Lord. I yearn to see You again with Your crown and sceptre and discus. Please show Yourself to me again in Your own four-armed form, O You of infinite forms.'

Krishna responded, 'Through My yogic power which I have shown you, you were able to see My cosmic form which is radiant, omnipresent and eternal. No one else has seen Me this way except you. One cannot get this vision through spiritual practices, by charitable gifts, performing ritual offerings, or by severe cleansing practices. You have seen the tremendous form of My greatness, but do not be afraid. Let go of your fear and, with a happy heart, see that other form of Mine.'

Having said this, Krishna reappeared in his human form, and the God of all calmed Arjuna's troubled mind.

Arjuna said, 'Now that I can see You in Your gentle human state, I can return to my own nature with peace in my heart.'

Krishna replied, 'You have now seen My Divine form that is so hard to see, for even the gods in heaven long to see what you have seen. Not by studying the scriptures, nor by living an austere life, nor through charitable ways, nor by making offerings to Me can I be seen as you have seen Me. Only by love and devotion to Me can people see Me, know Me and come to Me. Those who desire Me above all else, and completely devote themselves to Me, dedicating all that they do to Me, with no attachment to anything, and with love for all creation: it is they that in truth reach Me.'

12. Yoga of Devotion And the Path of Love

Arjuna asked, 'Who are the best yogis, those that worship You as visible in one form or another, or those that worship the invisible God?'

Krishna answered, 'Those who have their hearts set on Me, and lovingly worship Me with unshakeable faith when I am known in one form or another, are the perfect yogis. And those that worship Me as the Infinite, the Invisible, the Omnipresent, using all the powers of their spirit harmoniously to control their senses, and with the same loving mind for all, finding good in all beings – they reach in truth My very Self.

'But it is more difficult for those who focus their minds on the Imperceptible, because it is very hard for mortals to reach that goal. But for those whose very action is dedicated to Me, focused on Me, and who worship Me and meditate lovingly on Me with single-minded devotion, I deliver them free from the ocean of their samsaras, of life and death and rebirth.

'If you set your heart on Me, keep thinking about Me, concentrate your mind on Me, and think about who I am, then you will find that we are forever united. But if you are unable to rest your mind on Me, then seek to reach Me through the practice of yogic concentration. If you are not able to practise concentration, then dedicate all your work to Me. By dedicating all your actions to Me, you can also reach perfection. But if you cannot even do that, then take refuge in Me. Subdue your mind and give up any desire for personal rewards as the result of your actions.

'Concentration is better than mere practice, and meditation is better than concentration; but higher than meditation is to surrender lovingly the fruits of your actions, for this surrendering will bring you peace. The person who offers good will to all, who is friendly and compassionate, who does not feel separate from others, having no thoughts of "I" or "mine", who stays peaceful in pleasure and sorrow, and who is forgiving; this ever-contented yogi, who through meditation is steady in mind, who is controlled, and whose determination is strong; who offers her heart and mind to Me – this one is very dear to Me, loving Me with complete devotion.

'I love the person who is beyond excitement, anger and fear, neither agitated by the world nor a source of agitation. I love that devotee who is free from vain expectations, detached from personal desires, pure in mind, who works for God and not for himself, and is fair to all. I love those whose devotion has led them above the dualities, neither celebrating good fortune, nor running from pain, feeling neither joy nor hatred, grief nor desire.

'I love the person whose love is the same for herself as for her enemies and friends; whose mind stays balanced in honour or dishonour, who is beyond heat or cold, beyond pleasure and pain, and who is free from the chains of attachments. I love the person who gives equal weight to praise

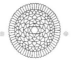

and blame, content with her lot in life, taking refuge in silence wherever she may be, whose mind is always steady, and whose heart is full of devotion.

'But the dearest to Me are those who have faith and love, and who regard Me as their Supreme goal, who hear My words of Truth, and who come to the waters of Everlasting Life.'

13. Yoga of Spirit and Matter

Aruna asked, 'Krishna, I would like to know more about Nature and the Self, the field and the one who knows the field, that which can be known and the wisdom or knowledge that knows it. What is the difference between the world and Divinity? Or the difference between one's worldly body and Godly Spirit?'

Krishna replied, 'I am the Self or Spirit in all bodies. People are enlightened and develop the deepest intuition when they understand the difference between the field, which is their physical body and everything else in the material world, and the knower of the field, which is their intelligence.

'I will tell you about the field – the world of Nature – and how changes take place in it. I will also show you who the knower is and tell you about his powers. This wisdom has been chanted by the rishis in many different ways through the ages.

'The field, Nature, originates in the Supreme Consciousness of Divinity. In the Natural world, this Consciousness separates into many physical and mental forces, which combine to make up the myriad things of the world. There are twenty-five components that make up the field, and the first is unmanifested Nature, the hidden seed from which both physical and spiritual things arise.

'From the unmanifested there arises in us the intellect,

which is the ability to discriminate between what is Real and what is not-Real, the true and the false. From having an intellect we become aware of being a singular creature, an "I" or ego. Working with the ego is the mind, which acts together with the senses to convey messages from Nature to the intellect. The mind works through the body's ten sense perceptions and mechanisms, which comprise the five perceptions: hearing, touch, taste, sight and smell, and the five organs of action: speech, hands, feet, and the reproductive and eliminative organs.

'The ten sense perceptions and mechanisms are attracted to five subtle essences in the world, which are called the objects of sense. These comprise: visible light waves, audible sound waves, tactile feelings, the tastes of flavour and the smell of odours and fragrances. Finally the mind organizes all of matter into the five basic elements of earth, water, air, fire and space. The last component of Nature is the most important and mysterious: it is prana, the life force, the Spirit, that breathes life into all of this matter. Arising within the field are desire and aversion, pleasure and pain, the collective organism of the body that holds all this together, intelligence and will.

'Those who know the world of Nature have humility and do not hurt others; they are forgiving and upright; they are devoted to their spiritual teacher; and they are pure, steady and have control of their minds. They are free from the lust of their senses and egoistic thoughts, and no longer identify with their own bodies and minds, or the field that continually undergoes the eternally changing cycles of birth, suffering, old age, disease and death.

'They have no personal attachments and whilst they still love their homes, families, husbands, wives, children or parents they no longer mistakenly identify themselves with them. They maintain a constant equanimity in pleasant or unpleasant events.

'Enjoying the yoga of steady devotion to Me, their hearts are full of pure love; they seek to be in quiet places, avoiding the noisy multitudes.

'They have a constant yearning to know the inner Spirit, and a vision of the true essence of Divine Knowledge which brings liberation: this is true wisdom. Seeking anything else is ignorance.

'Now I will tell you what you need to know to go beyond death to immortality: it is the supreme Brahman, without beginning, beyond what is and beyond what is not. He is everywhere, in every hand and every foot, every head, speaking through every mouth, hearing through every ear: He exists in all and He is. Brahman is devoid of senses yet His subtle powers perform the tasks of the senses. He is beyond all, yet he supports all. He is beyond the world of matter, and yet He has joy in this world. He is outside and within all things. He is far and He is near. He moves and yet He is still. He is invisible and cannot be seen. He is One in all, but it seems as if He were many, appearing to divide His Self into different creatures. He supports all beings: from Him comes destruction and from Him comes creation.

'Deep in the hearts of all beings is the Light of all lights, shining beyond all darkness. This is wisdom, the goal of all knowledge and what we need to know.

'So I have told you briefly now about the field, wisdom and what is to be known. When a person knows this he enters My Being. Know, Arjuna, that Nature – which is the field – and the knower – which is the Self, pure consciousness – are both without beginning; and know that the changes and power of Nature arise from Nature itself, as its forces combine and recombine to make new forms, shapes or actions.

'Nature is a web made of an infinite cycle of causes and effects leading one to another endlessly, and creating all actions in the universe. In us these causes work through the body, mind and the senses. Spirit is the source of all consciousness, able to experience pleasure and pain.

'The Spirit of man when integrated with Nature feels the ever-changing conditions of Nature. By clinging to pleasing experiences, the Spirit becomes lost to us, and this binds us to the cycle of birth and death.

'The Supreme Lord is present in all of us, watching over the games of our lives although unaffected by any of them. The yogi who in truth knows this Spirit and knows Nature with its changing conditions wherever she may be, has gone beyond karma and is free from the cycles of birth and death.

'Some people realize the truth through meditation, others through acquiring the knowledge of Jnana Yoga, others through Karma Yoga, the path of selfless service. There are also those who do not follow these paths, but hear from others about Self-realization and through pure devotion cross over beyond death to immortality.

'Whatever is born, whether it moves or is still, comes from the union between matter – the field – and the Spirit – the knower. Those who are able to see that the Spirit, that abides in us all, lives on when the body dies, have found the Truth. And when we see that the God in ourselves is the same God that exists in all that is, we do not hurt ourselves or others: in this way we reach the Supreme goal.

'Those that see the Truth understand that all actions everywhere are only the work of Nature and that Spirit does not perform actions: the body belongs to Nature and Spirit belongs to the Atman, the Spirit within. Those who understand Brahman can see that all creatures, although they appear separate, are truly only One: all emanating from Brahman and united in Brahman.

'The Self has no beginning and is free from changing conditions, and although it lives in the perishable body, it is deathless. It neither acts nor is affected by anything that is done.

'Just as the one sun lights up all things in this world, so

the Lord of the field – God – enlightens all creation. When the Self sees clearly and intuitively understands the difference between the field and the knower of the field, between the path of total freedom and being caught by Nature's illusions, then you have attained the Supreme wisdom.'

14. Yoga of the Three Forces of Nature

Krishna continued, 'I will now tell you in more detail about the Supreme Wisdom that has taken sages and saints to a state of Supreme perfection. Those who live by this wisdom have become part of Me: they are not reborn at the time of creation, nor do they die. It is I who places the seed of all births into the immense womb of Nature, and thus all beings are created. Everything that comes has Nature as his mother and Me as the Father that gave him life.

'The forces of Nature are three: sattva, the light, clear, and serene harmony of pure intelligence and goodness; rajas, the fiery restless energy of anger, hatred, greed and lust; and tamas, the darkness of dullness and inertia. Until final freedom is reached, these forces are clouds of matter darkening the light of the Spirit.

'Although the harmonious force is pure, giving light and health without obstructions, it still binds your mind through an attachment to happiness and knowledge. The restless active force is of the nature of passion, creating a thirst for acquiring worldly things and thus leading to the bondage of selfish attachment and compulsive behaviour. The dark lethargic force arises out of ignorance and deludes all creatures, binding them to sleepy dullness, carelessness and laziness.

'Sattva binds you to happiness, rajas binds you to incessant activity, while tamas leads to confused thinking and bad judgement. Sometimes sattva prevails over rajas and tamas, at other times rajas prevails over tamas and sattva, and at other times, tamas over sattva and rajas. The light, harmonious sattva is dominant when the light of wisdom shines from all the gates of the body. When the fiery rajas is dominant, we see greedy behaviour, busy activity, restlessness, discontentment and desire. When the dark tamas is dominant, there is a disinclination to act, ignorance, laziness, delusion and confusion.

'If your mind is in a predominantly sattvic state when the body dies, then your soul goes to the pure heaven of beings who know the Creator. If rajas predominates when a being dies, the soul will be reborn among those who are attached to action. And if it dies when tamas predominates, the soul is later reborn to parents who are deluded and ignorant of the Truth.

'Actions performed in a sattvic state result in wisdom and purity; actions performed in a rajasic state result in pain and greed; and those of a tamasic state result in neglect of duty, carelessness, ignorance and delusion of reality. Those who live mainly in sattva follow the path to a higher place, whilst those in rajas remain on the level path, and in tamas they lose ground and sink to the lower path.

'The yogis who understand that the forces of Nature are only the actors in the drama of life and can transcend Nature, attain the Supreme. When a yogi goes beyond the three forces of Nature which constitute her mortal body, she enters into immortality, free from the cycles of birth and death.'

Arjuna asked, 'How do we know the person who has passed beyond the three forces of Nature? How does she live? And how did she get past the three forces?'

Krishna replied, 'When Nature's qualities are present, these people neither attach to nor reject the light, activity or delusion that comes from the three forces. And when these qualities are not present, they do not miss them. They are aware that the forces of Nature are merely playing their part, so they are able to be unperturbed by changing conditions, remaining steady and unmoved. They dwell in their inner Selves, viewing pain and pleasure alike, seeing stones or gold or earth as one and the same, maintaining equanimity in the midst of pleasure and pain. They are beyond praise and blame and keep a steady and quiet mind. For them honour or disgrace is the same; and they have the same love for their enemies as for their friends. Surrendering all selfish actions, these people have gone beyond the three forces of Nature.

'And she whose never-failing love serves Me with the yoga of devotion, transcends the three forces and can be one with Brahman, the One. For I am the home of Brahman, the Immortal and unalterable never-failing fountain of everlasting life, dwelling in all as their Atman. I am the eternal truth and infinite joy.'

15. Yoga of the Supreme Self

Krishna said, 'There is a tree, the eternal tree, a sacred fig tree with its roots above close to God, and its branches suspended here on earth below. This tree's leaves are the holy scriptures, and those who understand this tree know the most sacred wisdom. Its branches spread from earth up to heaven and the three powers of Nature give them life. The tree's buds are the pleasures of the senses, and its roots stretch all the way down into this world, binding each person through selfish actions. The true nature of this tree and its changing form, its beginning and its end, and even its roots, cannot be seen through worldly awareness. But the wise can see its true nature if they cut down this deep-rooted tree with the sharp sword of non-attachment.

'There is a place from which they will never return. That

place is the goal. Look for this path by saying: 'I take refuge in that Eternal Spirit who is the Lord and source of all, the Absolute from whom the stream of creation came at the beginning. Those who are free from pride and ignorance, and who have conquered personal attachment, living in the Self, their true essence, with all selfish desires gone, and with equal steadiness in pleasure or pain, reach that eternal goal, the abode of eternity. In that place, the sun does not shine, the moon does not give light, and fire does not burn, because My radiance shines there: that is where I am. Once the individual soul achieves this ultimate enlightenment, they are forever with Me and never return to a separate existence.

A small part of My eternal Spirit takes the form of a living soul in this world and attracts Nature's forces. This soul draws around itself the five senses, with the mind as the sixth, since the mind and the senses are a part of Nature. When the Atman, the individual Self, enters and leaves a physical body, It takes with It the senses and the mind, just as the wind blows away the scent of perfume. The Atman, the Self, settles in the ears, nose, the senses of taste, touch and even the mind; so it is the Lord who actually experiences and enjoys the objects of the senses. Those who are deluded and unaware of the True Self within, do not realize who it is that leaves the body at the moment of physical death, nor are they aware of that living presence within themselves that gives life to the body, enjoys the senses, and experiences the powers of Nature. But those with intuitive insight can see and understand.

'Those seekers of yoga, with pure mind and heart, discover the Atman within themselves. Those who are neither pure nor wise never see Him, however hard they may strive. Know that the radiance of the sun that lights up the world, and the light of the moon and fire, all come from one Light which is My light. I come into the earth and with life-giving love and energy sustain all things on the earth. I am the life-giving sap that nourishes the world of plants. I am the fire of life that is in all breathing things. I am the heat in their digestive systems, that transforms food into strength. I am the in-breath and the out-breath. I am prana and apana, the living breaths of energy.

'And I am in the heart of all. With Me come memory and wisdom, and I also take them away. I am the knower and the knowledge of the *Vedas*, the holy scriptures, and the creator of the Vedanta, their end and essence. I am their goal. There are two Spirits in this world; one that is changeable and perishable, and the other that never changes and never dies. All created beings are perishable, but their Spirit is imperishable. But the highest Spirit is another: it is called the Spirit Supreme. He is the God of eternity who pervades and sustains the worlds. I am that Supreme Consciousness, beyond the perishable and beyond the imperishable. The enlightened beings see Me as the supreme Self. They know everything there is to know and worship Me with all their hearts.

'And so Arjuna, the pure, I have revealed the most secret doctrine to you. Anyone who has seen its light and understands this with all their heart becomes enlightened and wise. With this, there is nothing more to accomplish in life.'

16. Yoga of Heaven and Hell

Krishna said, 'Arjuna, these are the qualities and practices of people who will attain a Divine state: fearlessness; purity of heart, body and mind; steadfastly maintaining the yoga path of wisdom, generosity, control of the senses, a life of self-sacrifice, study of the holy scriptures, purification, integrity, non-violence, truthfulness, freedom from anger, serenity, without worldly attachments and desires, never speaking falsely or badly of others, compassion for all beings, peace from greedy cravings, gentleness, modesty, steadiness, full of energy, forgiving, courageous in adversity, with good-will and without hatred to anyone, and freedom from pride. These are the treasured characteristics of the person who is born with a Divine nature.

'Those qualities and practices destined for a person who is born to live in hell are: deceitfulness, arrogance, self-conceit, anger, cruelty and ignorance of the Truth. The Divine virtues bring freedom, whilst undesirable qualities imprison the soul. You, however, are born with the Divine attributes.

'There are two types of people in this world, those with predominantly Divine qualities, and those with predominantly undesirable ones. I have already told you at length of the Divine qualities, and I will now tell you of the undesirable ones. Heartless people do not know what is right and what is wrong. There is no purity or truthfulness in their hearts, and they do not behave well. They do not believe that there is a God, nor any truth or moral foundation in the world. And since they do not believe in a God of creation, they believe that birth is the result of lust and sex.

'Holding these distorted views and with so little intuitive understanding, these heartless people are the enemies of themselves and the world, bringing suffering and destruction. Their tortured souls are full of insatiable desires and they are full of hypocrisy, deceit, insolence and pride. In their delusion, they cling to their evil ideas and carry on their impure work. With their highest aim sensual enjoyment, believing fervently that this is all there is, they are weighed down with constant anxieties that stay with them until their death. Bound by vain hopes, anger and greed, they will do anything to amass as much wealth as they can to satisfy their cravings. They say, "Today I have this. Tomorrow I shall have that. This is mine and I will become even more wealthy. I have already killed that person and I will kill others. I am a lord; I enjoy life. I am successful, powerful and happy this way. I am rich and born of good stock. Who is there who can compare to me? I will pay for religious rituals, I shall give to charity, and take pleasure in my generosity."

'This is what they say in the darkness of their delusions. Misled by wrong thoughts, deluded and out of touch with reality, chained to the pleasure of their cravings, they sink into corruption and despair. Conceited and drunk with the pride of their wealth, they work against the Divine law as they ostentatiously make religious offerings. Full of arrogance and a selfish and insatiable lust for power, sex and wealth, these people hate Me: they hate Me in themselves and in others.

'Time after time I send these people to be reborn to the lowest and worst kind of parents. Each time, they are reborn in a lower life, unable to reach Me, sinking lower and lower into the path of hell. Hell has three gates of self-destruction: lust, anger and greed. Therefore, one should abandon these three. When a person is freed from these three doors of darkness, he can rise to the Path Supreme, the highest goal of life. But those who reject the world of the scriptures and follow the impulse of their desires do not reach perfection, or happiness and success. Let the Scriptures guide you as to what is right and what is wrong. Follow their words and do in this life the work that is to be done.'

17. Yoga of the Three-fold Faith

Arjuna asked, 'How do you regard people who do not follow the words of the scriptures, but offer sacrifices with sincere faith? What will their spiritual attainment be? Is the nature of their faith pure and serene, or fiery, active and energetic, or dark and inert?'

Krishna replied, 'There are three different kinds of faith

depending on a person's nature, which can be sattvic (light), rajasic (fiery), or tamasic (dark). Man is made of faith; he is as his faith. Those who are pure and sattvic by nature, worship one form of God or another; the restless and rajasic minds worship power and wealth; and those of tamasic darkness worship ghosts and spirits of the night.

'Those selfish and false people who choose severe ascetic practices that are not advised in the scriptures, are motivated by ego, lust, personal attachments and desires. They are fools who torture the powers of life in their bodies and also torture Me who lives within them. Know that their minds are in darkness. Those with the three differing qualities of faith also have differences over how they prefer their food, how they perform their duties, and how they follow their spiritual disciplines.

'People who are pure like food which is pure and healthy, giving them mental power, strength and long life: food which is tasty, comforting and nourishing. Those of a rajasic, restless and compulsive temperament prefer food which is acidic and sharp, very spicy, hot, bitter or very salty. Like the people who eat it, this food produces pain, grief, and disease. Those of a tamasic temperament, the dull and the lazy, choose food which is stale and tasteless, or food that has been left to rot overnight, impure and spoiled: food that is no longer nutritious.

'Sacrifice is sattvic and pure when it is offered for its own sake, without desire for reward, and offered with a pure and devoted mind in harmony with the holy law. However, any offering that is made with the expectation of reward, or ostentatiously, is not a pure sacrifice, and is of a rajasic quality. A sacrifice that is offered with no sincerity or faith, without the appropriate prayers and gifts, is a sacrifice of darkness and is tamasic.

'The body is harmonized with reverence for God, religious leaders, spiritual teachers and the wise; and also with purity, righteousness, chastity and non-violence. Harmony of speech comes with speaking truthfully, kindly, and pleasantly, as well as from reading aloud the sacred books. Harmony of the mind comes from tranquillity, gentleness, silence, loving kindness and a pure heart. To reach harmony of these three, these disciplines must be practised zealously and sincerely with no desire for reward, and with the mind controlled; this is real purity – sattvic.

'But false disciplines performed to gain respect, esteem and admiration are hypocritical and are rajasic; they are unstable, transient and uncertain. When these purification practices are performed in order to control, hurt or destroy someone else, or when self-control is self-torture with the mistaken belief that this is spiritually beneficial, these disciplines are then based on delusion and ignorance, and can be described as tamasic.

'A gift is pure when it is given from the heart to the right person at the right time, and without any expectation of return. But when it is given unwillingly, or with the expectation of something in return, then the gift is impure and is given in a tamasic state of dullness. And a gift given to the wrong person at the wrong time, without affection, or a gift that does not come from the heart and is given without due regard, is a gift of darkness.

'OM TAT SAT are the three words that represent the Supreme Consciousness from which everything else comes: spiritual wisdom, the scriptures and self-sacrifice. OM TAT SAT means THAT is the truth. Spiritual seekers chant OM when beginning spiritual disciplines, making devotional offerings and giving charity, as described in the holy scriptures. Those seeking enlightenment and liberation chant TAT as a reminder that their spiritual disciplines, devotional offerings and giving of charity are done without desire for reward, and are done with complete devotion to God. SAT means that which IS: what is good and what is true.

Chanting SAT blesses your activities. SAT also means constant faithfulness in sacrifice, self-discipline and selfless giving; and any action performed for the sake of the Divine. Any sacrifice offered, or gift given, or work done without faith, is not worthwhile because it is ASAT, without truth, and nothing worthwhile will come of it in this life or in the life to come.'

18. Yoga of Freedom through Renunciation: Knowing, Acting and Loving

Arjuna said, 'Please tell me again about the essence of renunciation and the essence of surrender, non-attachment.'

Krishna replied, 'Renouncing all selfish works is renunciation, and letting go of desire for the rewards of your work is non-attachment and surrender. Some of the wise ones say that all actions should be renounced, since action disturbs contemplation, but others believe that works of sacrifice, selfless giving, self-discipline and purification should not be renounced.

'I will now tell you about the essence of non-attachment. There are three levels of non-attachment. Self-sacrifice, purification, selfless giving and self-discipline should not be given up; they must be continued because these actions purify the mind and make you wise. But these actions must also be performed with no expectation of return or reward. It is not correct to neglect to do the work that we need for our spiritual path.

'To give this up would be to fall into a tamasic delusion of darkness. Avoiding action because you are afraid of physical discomfort and pain is rajasic, and brings no spiritual benefit. Performing your duties because it is the right thing to do, surrendering selfishness and any desire of reward, brings calm, peace and the pure sattvic state.

'In this way, letting go of all personal attachments, you will be filled with purity and peace; and work, whether pleasant or painful, is a joy. It is not possible for anyone to let go of action completely, but what we can do is to let go of the hope of a reward: this is true detachment. Those who are still attached, and who act out of selfishness, will experience three types of consequences to their actions: unpleasant, pleasant and mixed. But those who renounce desire and attachment are able to transcend their karma.

'I shall now explain about the five factors that the scriptures say make every action happen. The first is the body without which there is no action; the second is the ego, the doer of the action; the third is the sense organs; the fourth is the motion or energy that performs the action; and the fifth is the various aspects of God that correspond with different parts of the body and fate.

'Whatever a person does, whether it is good or bad in thought, word or deed has these five elements that bring about each action. This is how things are. The person who does not understand this is a person of clouded vision: he believes that he makes things happen rather than that things happen through him, or he believes that it is the Atman, the individual Spirit, that acts.

'The person who is no longer chained by selfishness and the ego-driven sense of being separate, is not tainted by his actions. Therefore, although it may seem that he kills his enemies, he is in fact not the doer and is not bound by those actions.

'When we have the idea of action, there are three elements: knowledge, what is to be known, and the one who knows. The three components of action are the means (the part of the body we use to perform the action), the action itself, and the individual who performs the action.

'Looking at these three components from the perspective of the three forces of Nature, I shall tell you about the three types of knowledge, the three types of action and the three types of doers. The sattvic person of pure knowledge can see the Eternal Reality that is in everything and everyone: the indivisible oneness of all creatures of the universe. The rajasic person with a restless mind sees everything, and all the various creatures, as very different and separate from each other. Seeing one part of the whole and mistaking it for all there is, is tamasic knowledge, which is ignorant.

'An action that is done unselfishly, with a peaceful and devoted mind, without love or hatred, and with no desire for reward, is a pure sattvic action. The rajasic action of a restless mind is done with the intent of personal reward to satisfy the ego, or with the feeling that the action is an effort. And the tamasic work of darkness is done with a confused mind, without considering the possible consequences of harm to himself or another, and is blind to his own capacity to carry out the action.

'Sattvic doers see it all as the work of the Divine and see themselves as instruments of Divinity, and as such are free from attachment to rewards, and free of the egoistic feeling of separateness, yet full of enthusiasm, not affected by success or failure. The rajasic doers act primarily out of personal desire to reap the rewards of actions, or out of greed, violence or impurity: they become joyous or despondent with success or failure. Tamasic doers do things inattentively with stubbornness, laziness and lethargy and an unsteady mind, cheating others maliciously.

'Now, Arjuna, I will teach you about the three degrees of understanding and the three types of will from the perspective of each of Nature's three forces. These are the signs of sattvic understanding, of pure wisdom: knowing when and when not to act; knowing what is the right thing to do and what is wrong; knowing what is fear and what is courage; knowing the paths of bondage and liberation.

Rajasic understanding, impure wisdom, has no clear vision of what is right and what is wrong, what should be done and what should not be done. Tamasic understanding is shrouded in darkness, seeing what is wrong as right, and has a distorted view of everything.

'In yoga meditation the movements of the mind and breath of life are pure, steady and strong; and with this sattvic will comes the control of the mind, prana (life energy), and the senses. The rajasic will strongly desires wealth, power, prestige and sense pleasures. The signs of a tamasic will are born of ignorance, a lack of purpose and a lack of strength, filled with laziness, fear, self-pity, depression and conceit.

'Now, Arjuna, I shall tell you about the three kinds of pleasure, one of which is the pleasure of steadily following the right path that leads to the end of all pain and sorrow. Sattvic happiness is the serenity and clarity of mind that comes from Self-realization: bitter poison at the beginning and sweet nectar at the end. Rajasic happiness is the opposite: nectar at the beginning and poison at the end, because it is a temporary pleasure only, as the senses come into contact with worldly objects that they desire. Tamasic happiness is both at its beginning and at its end a delusion of the soul that comes from the dullness of excess sleep, laziness or carelessness.

'There is no being on earth nor Gods in the heavens who are free from these three powers of Nature. In fact, Arjuna, the qualities in one's own nature determine the appropriate role and duty for each person, whether scholar or priest, leader, warrior, tradesperson or labourer. By nature the priests or seers tend to be peaceful, serene, self-controlled, self-disciplined, forgiving, and loving, having faith in the Eternal and filled with spiritual wisdom and empirical knowledge. Leaders or warriors are by nature courageous, fearless, resourceful and generous, with firmness of mind and determination not to flee from a battle, with strong leadership qualities. The tradespeople by their nature tend to move towards farming, cattle rearing and business. The working people by their nature work with, for and in the service of society.

'We can all achieve perfection by doing what is right for us to do, and joyfully following the work that is our duty. We attain this perfection when our work is our calling, and then we worship God, from whom all things come, and who is in all. It is better to follow your own path imperfectly, than to follow someone else's path, even if it is greater than yours. When a person does the work that God gives him, he is free from sin. We must never give up the duties of our own nature even if the results are sometimes blemished. Nothing that we ever do is perfect, just as fire produces smoke.

'The person whose mind and intellect is no longer attached to anything, and who has subdued and gone beyond his selfish ego and the desire for pleasure, rises to a state of perfection and is free from the bondage of karma. Now I will tell you again how it is possible to reach Brahman, the Supreme state of wisdom. To become one with Brahman you must have pure understanding, become self-restrained with firm control of your senses and passions, let go of the sights, tastes, and sounds of the world, and go beyond likes and dislikes. You must dwell in the solitude of silence, continually engaging in yogic meditation, eating sparely and controlling your thoughts, words and actions. And when your selfishness, lust, anger and pride have gone, and you free yourself from the thought "This possession is mine", and you are calm and peaceful within yourself, then you are worthy to experience oneness with the Absolute.

'When you merge in the Brahman, with peace in your heart, you neither grieve nor suffer the anxiety of personal desires. When your love is one for all creation, you rise to a state of supreme devotion to Me, the Lord. With such complete and pure devotion, you shall know Me in truth, who I am and what I am. And when you know Me in truth you can enter into my Being. By taking refuge in Me, all your actions are serving Me. Fully concentrated on Me, you will come home to Me in the imperishable state of eternity. Offer every thought and act to Me, the Supreme, and take refuge in the yoga of understanding, to know what is real and what is not. Keep your mind fixed on Me, for it is by loving God that you will rise from the human to the Divine. If your mind remains fixed on Me, then with My grace, you shall over-come all obstacles. But if you get caught up in your egoism and do not hear My words, then you will perish.

'If you make the conscious decision, out of fear and self-conceit, not to fight the battle, this decision is not founded on your true nature, and your unconscious will compel you to fight. Arjuna, since you are bound by karma, the forces of your past life and actions, you will have to act in confor-mity with your nature, even if in your delusion you think you do not want to. God dwells in the hearts of all beings, Arjuna: and by His own power of illusion whirls them around as if they were puppets in a play of shadows. With all your heart take shelter with Him. Then by His grace you will obtain a Supreme peace which is your eternal home.

'I have now taught you the most profound and precious knowledge, the secret of secrets. Think about it deeply, reflect on it, and then do whatever you wish to. I will now tell you for the last time My highest teaching, the mystery of all mys-teries; I tell you this because your devotion to Me is so strong, and you are so very dear to Me. Focus your mind on Me always, dedicate every action to Me, devote your heart to Me and surrender yourself to Me. Then you shall come to Me. I assure you of this truth because you are so precious to Me. Give up all your duties and come to Me alone for shelter, where there is no grief or sorrow. I will free you from the bondage of your sins and guilt.

'You must never speak about these things to anyone who lacks self-discipline, or has no love, or does not want to hear about Me, or who argues against Me. But he who teaches this secret doctrine to those that have love for Me, and who himself has Supreme love, in truth he shall come directly to Me. For there cannot be any person who does greater work for Me, nor any one on earth who is dearer to Me. Those who study this sacred dialogue with deep sincerity worship Me with wisdom and devotion. And those who only listen to these words with faith and acceptance are freed from evil, and enter the happy realms of the righteous.

'Arjuna, have you heard all this with a focused and clear mind? Has the darkness of your delusion finally been destroyed?'

Arjuna replied, 'Yes, my delusion has been destroyed, and my power and joy have come back to me. By Your grace, I am free of doubts and my faith is firm. I will now follow my path that has been chosen by You: Your will be done.'

Here ends the dialogue between the supreme Lord Krishna and the noble-souled Prince Arjuna. Their words have filled our souls with awe and wonder. By the grace of the poet Vyasa, we have heard these profound secrets of yoga wisdom directly from Krishna, the Lord of Yoga. As we remember this marvellous and holy dialogue between Krishna and Arjuna, we are overcome with joy. And whenever we remember the astonishing form of Krishna, the vision of glory of the God of all, we rejoice again and again. Whenever you come upon Krishna, the Lord of Yoga, and Arjuna, the great archer – Divinity and humanity – you too will find victory, happiness and beauty in the battle of life. Have faith in this.

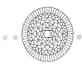

III

The *Yoga Sutras*

1. Yoga Is Control of the Mind

◆ Here are the true teachings of yoga.
◆ Yoga means to control and still the swirling currents of thoughts in the mind. If you can control the thoughts that arise, and still them completely, you are able to observe the world clearly and directly without the distortions of the ego. The ability to discipline the chattering mind is what takes us to the state of yoga.
◆ When the turbulence stops and the lake of the mind becomes clear and still, our true essence, our Self, is reflected. Then the Self can abide in its own true nature. This is the goal, this is what we want to attain.
◆ When we fail to still our minds we mistakenly identify our Self with the activities of the mind, and become lost in our thoughts. We lose the true sense of who we are because we have lost sight of our true essence, our real inner Self.

2. The Five Kinds of Mental Activity

◆ There are five kinds of mental activity, which lead us to either happiness or misery.
◆ The five kinds of mental activity are understanding or right knowledge, misconception or error, fantasy and verbal delusion, deep sleep and memory.
◆ Understanding comes from first-hand experience of our senses – for example, we know when we touch something hot, we burn. Or by inference, that every flame would burn, or by believing some trustworthy authority. Our senses provide us with true understanding only when we harbour no element of delusion.
◆ Misconception occurs when our knowledge of something is not based on its true form and we misinterpret what

we perceive. There is a classic example of this in yoga literature: in the twilight a man sees a coiled rope on the earth and mistakes it for a snake. Fear overtakes him and he hurls himself into a ditch, landing on a scorpion which bites him.

♦ Fantasy is knowledge based on words that have no objective existence. Verbal delusion arises when words do not correspond to reality and we arrive at untrue conclusions.

♦ Dreamless deep sleep is a wave of thought about nothingness. When we sleep deeply we have the thought of having no thought. It becomes a time lapse that we are only conscious of in retrospect, when we awake.

♦ Memory is when perceived objects, thoughts and feelings are not forgotten and return to consciousness. Memories are created by impressions on the mind that surface at a later time, while dreams are memories that come to the surface when we sleep. The thought waves that we experience when we sleep cause ripples in the mind and we experience these as dreams.

♦ These are the five activities of the mind that must be regulated to make the mind still and quiet and allow inner peace to shine through.

♦ We gain control over the mind's turbulence by persevering in our yoga practice and by not allowing our minds to attach to objects of desire.

♦ To reach any permanent control of thought waves we must continually practise steadying the mind. This practice becomes firmly grounded and established when we engage in it seriously and diligently over a long and uninterrupted period of time.

♦ Non-attachment is when we can completely let go and free ourselves from the desire for things we have seen or heard of, whether worldly or spiritual.

♦ When we discover and love our true Self, our real essence or Spirit, and find such peace and bliss that we no longer have any worldly desires, we have reached the highest level of non-attachment: at this point we feel love for every living thing. It is not that the qualities of the outer world have disappeared, but they have simply lost their powers of attraction.

3. The Eight Limbs of Yoga Practice

◆ When we regularly practise the eight limbs of yoga, our impurities dwindle away and there dawns the light of wisdom leading to intuitive understanding.

◆ The eight limbs of yoga are:
  ◆ yama – self-restraint
  ◆ niyama – personal observance
  ◆ asana – postures
  ◆ pranayama – breath control
  ◆ pratyahara – withdrawing our minds from sense objects
  ◆ dharana – concentration
  ◆ dhyana – meditation
  ◆ samadhi – contemplation and absorption in the Self

4. Yama and Niyama

◆ Yama or self-restraint consists of non-violence, honesty, not stealing, sexual moderation, and not being greedy.

◆ The rules of yama are basic rules of conduct. They should be practised regularly without concern for time, place or circumstance.

◆ The niyamas or personal observances consist of purity, contentment, discipline, the study of spiritual books and devotion to our personal God.

◆ When we are disturbed by negative thoughts, we must

cultivate positive ones to counteract them, developing an ability to control the negative.

♦ When we think or act in a negative way we have to understand that these actions or thoughts come from our own impatience, greed or anger; and the consequences of these actions and thoughts bring pain to ourselves and others, and are based on ignorance. Therefore it is important for us to cultivate positive thoughts and actions.

♦ When we are in the presence of someone who is established in non-violence, they radiate a feeling of calm and serenity.

♦ The actions of someone who really respects the truth will be both powerful and perfectly effective.

♦ When we are completely free from stealing and greed and contented with what we have, then through that serenity, wealth can come.

♦ The more sexually moderate we are, the more vitality we have.

♦ When we can persevere on the path neither to desire, acquire nor accept worldly things that we do not really need, we gain a deep understanding of the meaning of life.

♦ Purity protects our own body and brings us into non-physical relationships with others.

♦ First we need to understand and listen to our body's inherent wisdom, and then our hearts can become pure as well. We become more cheerful, have better concentration, more control over our senses and are more able to realize our Self.

♦ As a result of our contentment, we gain supreme happiness.

♦ When we get rid of our impurities, a disciplined life brings perfection and mastery over our body and senses.

♦ By studying spiritual writings, we are able to commune with our personal God.

♦ As a result of our devotion to God, we reach samadhi. By

dedicating the results of our work to God, and by always working with right means towards right ends, working to the best of our knowledge and ability at any particular moment, we may gradually achieve wisdom and non-attachment.

5. Asanas, Pranayama and Pratyahara

◆ The asanas or postures must be steady and comfortable.
◆ We are able to sit comfortably by meditating on the infinite, thereby lessening our natural tendency to become restless.
◆ If you make your posture firm and comfortable, you are no longer affected by life's dualities: praise and blame, heat and cold, wealth and poverty, and so on.
◆ Once we have been able to sit comfortably, we have to control our inhalation and exhalation. This is pranayama.
◆ The phases of breathing are inhalation, exhalation and retention. Noticing them in space, time and number, we are able to make our breath more harmonious, deeper and more subtle.
◆ As we enter into a deeper meditation on the source of the breath, the pauses between each inhalation and exhalation automatically lengthen.
◆ As a result we are able to discover our inner light and our perception becomes clearer. Then our mind becomes able to concentrate.
◆ When our mind is withdrawn from sense objects, the sense organs also withdraw themselves from their respective objects and are said to imitate the mind. This is known as pratyahara.
◆ Then we have complete mastery over our senses.

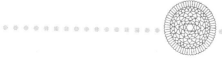

6. Discovering the Highest Knowledge

♦ Concentration is focusing the mind on one place, object or idea. Concentration on one thing is a discipline to train the mind, and it is the beginning of meditation.

♦ Meditation is the continuous awareness of that one object.

♦ We reach samadhi or absorption when we are meditating and the true nature of the object is clear and not distorted by our mind.

♦ When we are able to focus our mind for a prolonged period with concentration, meditation and contemplation, we are able perfectly to master our mind.

♦ When we have managed to master our mind and senses in this way, we are able to see the light of the highest knowledge.

7. The Last Three Limbs: Concentration, Meditation, Samadhi

♦ We have to accomplish this practice in stages.

♦ These last three limbs of yoga – concentration, meditation and absorption – are more internal than the first five limbs. When we compare these three limbs with the first five, they are all more internal, but when we compare them with the furthest and highest state of samadhi, we see that Samadhi is the real internal work.

♦ When we are able consciously to control the mind so that we no longer have any thoughts or visions, we can start to transform the mind to a state of stability.

♦ When we continue to regulate the waves of thoughts, the mind becomes calmer.

♦ When the distractions in our mind disappear and our mind becomes one-pointed, our mind becomes focused and absorbed.

- When the mind stays with the same object for a short period of time, it is called concentration; for a longer period, meditation; for a further time, lower samadhi; and finally, the highest samadhi.
- Even when we are experienced in contemplation and can make the mind peaceful and focused, it can still become disrupted because of thoughts arising from earlier states of mind that we had experienced.

8. Two Different Kinds of Concentration and Meditation

- Concentration and meditation upon a single object like a flame, or an abstract idea like a colour, follow a four-staged path or process: examining its outer aspect, reflection on its subtle inner essence, joyful peace in contemplation of it and a pure clear sense of just being.
- A second kind of meditation is when there is no object or idea to concentrate on, only consciousness itself. In this state, old and latent thoughts come up as ideas and images; these are like burnt seeds, the smallest seeds of old impressions still embedded in consciousness. In this state the old and buried seeds can still float into the conscious mind and pull you back into worldly turmoil.
- This state of meditation is reached by constantly examining the thoughts that arise, through the practice of non-attachment. The ultimate state we are aiming for is called samadhi where there is only pure awareness and nothing else: all ego feeling is gone, and the seeds of past impressions have lost their power. This samadhi gives us total liberation.
- Two kinds of people can attain the samadhi of pure awareness without an object: those who have attained the highest goal of liberation in an earlier life and have

returned to earth to help others, and those who are at a superior level, born full of wisdom, high intelligence and compassion.

◆ For others, the samadhi of pure awareness can be found through faith, strength, memory, or by deep understanding.

◆ Success in samadhi varies according to the means used to achieve it, whether gentle, moderate or intense. Success can come quickly to the keen and intent practitioner.

9. Devotion to a Personal God

◆ Another way to attain samadhi is through devotion to a personal God. A personal God is the source of all our knowledge. This God is our personal spiritual guide, our guardian.

◆ A personal God is a supreme spiritual being who is untouched by ignorance and free from all causes of suffering: free from desires and from karma: actions, and their consequences.

◆ Our personal God is all-knowing and is Himself the complete knowledge of the cosmos.

◆ Unconditioned by time, He is the original Teacher, and is the Teacher of all teachers.

◆ The sound which we use to express God is OM, the most sacred syllable.

◆ Reciting OM as a mantra while meditating on its meaning will lead to its full understanding.

10. The Obstacles to Truth

◆ Following these practices, we gradually clear away the obstacles in our minds that obscure the truth. We are able to turn inwards and uncover the true Self, our real essence.

◆ There are nine obstacles of the mind: illness, mental laziness, doubt, lack of enthusiasm, carelessness, delusion, craving objects, becoming disheartened due to lack of progress, and unsteadiness of mind.

◆ These mental distractions are accompanied by sorrow, depression, physical restlessness and disturbed breathing.

◆ All these distractions and obstacles can be removed by the disciplined practice of the technique of one-pointed concentration on a single truth or principle.

II. Calming the Mind

◆ The mind can be calmed by cultivating four important attitudes: an attitude of friendliness towards those who are happy, compassion towards the unhappy, delight and joy for the virtuous, and an indifference to those who do wrong.

◆ The mind can also be calmed through the control of the in-breath, retention of the breath and slow release of the out-breath. Where the mind goes, breath and prana follow. When the mind is concentrated and still, the breath slows to a stop and there is an automatic retention of the breath, without effort. This is the pause at the end of both the inhalation and the exhalation. You can discover this for yourself in deep meditation.

◆ Concentrating on subtle sense perceptions can also bring steadiness to the mind. If you concentrate your awareness on the tip of your nose, after a time you will notice an increased sense of smell; concentrating awareness on the tip of the tongue will give a heightened sense of taste.

◆ Concentrating on your inner light steadies the mind. Your Eternal Self can be found in the brilliant inner light radiating from your heart chakra, the energy centre of your heart. Seeing that supreme light within takes you beyond all anxieties, fear and worry.

♦ Or you can concentrate on a great teacher's mind and heart, one who has given up all worldly desires and has realized his Self.

♦ Or by concentrating on an experience that you had during a dream or in sleep. Sometimes when we sleep we dream of Divine beings; meditating on these Divine beings will bring us calm.

♦ Mental tranquillity can also come from meditating on anything that we find spiritually elevating.

♦ Control of the mind can then extend from the most minute particle to the vast magnitude of the great universe itself.

12. Four Kinds of Samadhi

♦ When the fluctuations of our minds subside, and the mind becomes clear and balanced like a jewel, the object of our concentration can then be reflected. We can concentrate on an object, such as a flame, or an organ of perception, like the eye, or an abstract idea, like the sense of ego. A state of fusion or identity between the Self and the object of concentration is known as samadhi. The mind is completely absorbed and loses itself in the object or idea of meditation.

♦ Samadhi with deliberation is when we consciously identify the object of concentration by its name, shape and our knowledge of it.

♦ Samadhi without deliberation is a higher stage where we identify the object of our concentration with only our intuitive inner knowledge of the object. We are able to still our reactions to the object and focus on it as it truly is without any preconceived ideas.

◆ There are also two other samadhis: reflective and non-reflective, when the object of concentration is a subtle one.

◆ When we concentrate reflectively on finer and more subtle objects such as the ego, or the correct vision of reality, we understand that the object is limitless and as such can trace it back to its very source.

◆ These kinds of samadhi are said to be accompanied by the small seeds of desire and attachment. The ultimate goal has not yet been reached. Even when we have acquired these states, we can still be seduced by our desires because the impressions of them remain latent in our consciousness. This is why we have to meditate with a pure mind.

◆ When we reach non-reflective samadhi the mind becomes clear and serene, and the clear light of our true inner Self shines out. This is absolute awareness, in which the mind is pervaded by true knowledge and understanding. We become our deepest knowledge, the wisdom of inner truth.

◆ This special truth is totally different from the knowledge we gain from hearing a lecture, or reading scriptures or from reasoning. This is the higher knowledge that can only be understood without the mind. Transcending the mind and revealing the knowledge of your inner essence is Self-realization – the ancient teachings of the yogis.

◆ The impressions made on the mind from this samadhi of absolute awareness remove all other past impressions, which disappear. We now understand our true nature and cannot return to an earlier state of ignorance.

◆ When even this impression is wiped out so that there are no more thought waves remaining in the mind, we enter the state of samadhi without deliberation. This is a state in which our awareness is also our being and our being is complete peace and joy.

13. The Obstacles to Liberation

◆ The practice of yoga also involves the study of spiritual writings and the resulting discipline of self-reflection allows us to let go of our personal concerns and to rely on a higher power. Self-discipline is an aid to spiritual progress, whereas self-torture is an obstacle.

◆ The aim of this practice is to cultivate the power of concentration and to remove the obstacles to enlightenment that are the cause of all our suffering.

◆ These five obstacles – the causes of our suffering – are present as part of our personality. They are ignorance, egoism, attachment to worldly things, hatred and the desire to cling to life.

◆ Ignorance is the source of the other four obstacles. Ignorance is a mistaken perception of life, when we mistake the unreal for the real, the impermanent for the permanent, the impure for the pure, the painful for the pleasant and the non-self as the true Self.

◆ The ego is the confusion of misidentifying our body, mind and senses as our true Self.

◆ Attachment is the consequence of pleasure, while aversion is the consequence of pain. We attach ourselves to objects of pleasure because we think they will make us happy, forgetting that true happiness is already within us as the true Self. Aversion is another form of bondage: we are tied to what we hate or fear.

◆ The desire to cling to life, the survival instinct, is inherent in both the ignorant and the learned.

◆ In meditation we are able to understand these obstacles

by seeing how our mind works, and we are able to clear them away.

◆ Even when we have overcome these obstacles in their fully developed form, there is inevitably a tiny remnant left. These remnants are finally destroyed when the mind traces them back to their origin in the ego, leading to samadhi.

14. Karmic Impressions

◆ Behaviour that is caused by these obstacles always leave impressions in the mind. Actions always bring reactions; causes lead to effects, which in turn become causes in endless karma. These always reveal themselves in some form or another, in this life or in future lives.

◆ Our karma determines the span of each life and how much we experience of pleasure or pain. The individual Soul always continues to evolve through time and space. We may even be reborn into the body of an animal.

◆ If you have done good things you experience pleasure and happiness; if wrong things, suffering.

15. Anguish and Its Avoidance

◆ The person who is spiritually aware sees all of life's experiences as painful. Even the enjoyment of present pleasure is painful since we already fear its loss. Past pleasure is also painful because we experience sharp cravings for it to come again. And how can happiness last if it depends on our moods, given that our moods are always changing as one or another of Nature's forces seize control of the mind?

◆ But it is possible to avoid suffering that has not yet come our way. Our pain comes because of the confusion between our inner Self who observes and the objects of Nature that we perceive.

16. The Self and Nature

- All objects of experience are composed of the three forces of Nature: clarity, activity and inertia. From these three the whole universe has evolved, together with the mind and the senses, and all objects perceived, such as the physical elements. The universe exists so that we can experience it, learn from it, and become liberated. We have to learn Nature's lessons.
- Nature is so diverse and multiform, and has so many dimensions, that most of us are able to see only the obvious ones, while some of us can discern the more subtle, and very few are able to see the extremely fine.
- The Self as pure awareness can only observe and not act. It uses the mind to experience Nature but remains unaltered itself.
- What we see exists only for us, the Self that observes.
- Once the intent of the Self is fulfilled, what was seen no longer exists for the Self. But what was seen still exists in Nature to serve others.
- Although the confusion of the Self and Nature is not correct, because spirit and matter are different, their union gives us the opportunity to discover the distinct nature of each – our inner essence and Nature and its powers.
- The cause of this confusion of Self and Nature is ignorance. This confusion only exists when we are ignorant of the true Self, and assume that our ego is our Self, and allow it to join with Nature.
- When ignorance disappears, there is no confusion of Self and Nature. The absence of confusion brings serenity. As

ignorance disappears gradually, the perception of reality grows ever clearer. When we are clear-sighted, we begin to feel serene and peaceful, and become liberated.

◆ When we are able to develop a lucid mind that see things objectively and positively, ignorance and confusion go. Wisdom dawns. We awaken our knowledge of the Self until no trace of illusion remains.

17. The Emergence of Wisdom

◆ The wisdom that emerges has seven stages.
These stages are:

i.   becoming aware of the desires that cause our suffering and knowing that the source of all spiritual wisdom is hidden within us.

ii. recognizing and removing the desires that cause suffering; when we turn our minds inwards to our inner essence, our attachments and aversions lose their power.

iii. understanding the mind fully, and with that neutral mind gaining cosmic understanding.

iv. when we understand Nature and its workings then we have a sense that there is no longer anything we have to do.

v.   once we know that there is nothing more to be done, then our minds become humble and simple and are free of impressions. We are liberated because we understand our real nature, our essence.

vi. then the stored-up impressions within the mind, and the forces of Nature, fall away forever.

vii. when we reach the final stage we are in a state of eternal existence in union with our Self. We no longer identify with our minds and bodies, but have reached samadhi.

18. The Ever-changing World

◆ In the state of higher samadhi, our minds are beyond any changes arising from thoughts. It makes no difference whether these thoughts are of different kinds, if they vary in intensity, or if they refer to different periods of time.

◆ Every object has its characteristics, and always has the possibility to change, either in the past, the present or in the future.

◆ Different situations create different changes. There are only two fundamental parts to the universe: being and change. If we learn to adapt to change, we will suffer less.

19. The Powers of the Mind

◆ By concentrating, meditating and reaching a state of samadhi, we can understand the past and the future.

◆ In this state of samadhi, if we can separate the sound of a word from both its meaning and our perception of it (three individual processes that are usually fused together), we can use this to reach an understanding of all sounds that we speak.

◆ If we concentrate, meditate on and absorb a thought that we have had for some time, we can gain insight into experiences that affected us in this life or in our past lives, and understand where our own conditioning comes from.

◆ When we can master the contents of our mind, we can know what someone else is thinking about, but we cannot know the motives behind their thoughts.

◆ When we master our physical bodies and appearance, allowing us to dissociate an observer's gaze on us, we make ourselves invisible, and the sounds that we utter are no longer heard.

- There are two kinds of karma: the kind that manifests quickly and the kind that manifests slowly. If we master the understanding of both of these, and also of our death, we may know the exact moment of our passing.
- When we can master friendliness, compassion and other such feelings, we can develop the power of these qualities.
- With perfect concentration on the strength of an elephant or some other strong animal, we can become strong like them.
- The mind must submerge itself into the light inside the heart in order for us to understand the subtleties and underlying causes that are buried beneath our habits and past life influences.
- When we have complete concentration on the sun, we gain knowledge of the entire solar system. If on the moon, we gain knowledge of the arrangement of the stars, and if on the pole star, we know the movement of the stars.

20. The Knowledge of the Body and Prana

- When we have complete concentration on the energy centre in the navel, the Manipura Chakra, we come to know the constitution of the body.
- Concentration on the pit of the throat, the Visuddha Chakra, takes away hunger and thirst.
- Perfect concentration on spinal alignment makes us stable.
- Complete concentration on the spiritual light at the crown of the head, the Sahasrara Chakra, makes us able to see celestial beings.
- Or we may gain psychic powers through the intuitive state we reach from living a life of purity.

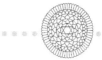

- Complete concentration on the heart gives us knowledge of the mind.
- We have to discern the difference between knowing our inner Self and our intellect. When we reach a state of perfect concentration on the Self, we can start to understand it. This way we can tell the difference between earthly pleasure and inner joy.
- With that understanding of the Self, we develop intuitive powers of hearing, touch, sight, taste and smell.
- These powers are obstacles in meditation but are effective powers in worldly life.
- If you have managed to separate your Self from your mind, and your mind from your body, you are able to enter another person's body and to cause it to move or to do what you wish.
- When we are able to control the nerve currents that govern the lungs and the upper part of the body, we have a feeling of lightness and ease as this energy rises.
- Mastering the force which regulates the various functions of our vital energy, we surround our bodies with a blaze of light.
- Mastery of the relationship between our ears and the space around us gives us the ability to have supernatural powers of hearing: we truly hear what is being said.
- Mastering the relationship between our body and space, we become very light and are able to fly.
- When our mental activity is no longer influenced by outside things and the veil that covers our internal light is removed, we become liberated.
- Complete concentration on the five elements we can perceive (earth, fire, water, air and space), and the understanding of them in relation to our own bodies, can give us perfect health.
- When we can master these five elements, we are able to

acquire powers to alter our weight, our size, our control over the environment, and so on . . .

◆ Perfection of our bodies means beauty, grace, strength and being solid as a diamond.

◆ Perfect mastery of the sense organs is very difficult to reach and maintain while they are linked to the three forces of Nature and their constant changes. However, through meditation and deep concentration we are able to understand our perceptions, the perceived objects, the perceiving entity, and its reference to our Self and our intent.

◆ As a result, the body has the power to move as fast as the mind, the ability to function without using the sense organs, and complete mastery of Nature, the primal cause.

21. Pure Awareness

◆ When we have reached a state of inner stability, there is still further to go; and as we recognize the difference between having our field of consciousness at peace and the state of absolute awareness, we reach a state of omniscience and omnipotence.

◆ The yogi who has held these psychic powers of omnipotence and omniscience within his grasp, and yet has been able to renounce them, rejecting the ultimate temptation of the ego, is freed from bondage and attains liberation.

◆ When we are tempted by invisible beings in high places, we must not be allured or flattered, because if we do we are in danger of being caught out once again by our ignorance.

◆ When we can perfectly master being present in the moment, we gain intuitive understanding.

◆ So we become able, with the spiritual value of this power

of intuition, to be able to distinguish between the Self and non-Self, between the essence within and outward appearance, however deceptive that may be.

♦ This intuitive understanding can relate to any object at any level. Such knowledge is infinite; it is within eternity, and is timeless.

♦ When all the thought waves in our minds have been stilled, the mind holds nothing but pure undifferentiated awareness. The pure still mind and the Self are the same. There is eternal peace and eternal joy.

22. The Law of Karma

♦ We can cultivate psychic powers through practices that were performed in previous lives, or by means of drugs, reciting mantras like OM, ascetic discipline or complete concentration and meditation.

♦ Evolution is a natural phenomenon that occurs from within and is not caused by external influences.

♦ Good and bad deeds do not directly cause natural evolution. They merely remove the obstacles in the way, just as a farmer breaks down a dam or opens sluice gates, to allow water to flow freely. The water is already there and flows into the field by the natural force of gravity. In the same way we all have perfection inside us, only we have to remove the obstacles, so the flow of awareness will be continuous and the water can reach its source.

♦ The only mind that is free from all karmic impressions is one that has been purified through meditation.

♦ The karma of the yogi is neither bad nor good, while the karma of others is either good, bad or mixed.

♦ In any particular life, our condition is determined by the balance of our karmas. Only the tendencies appropriate to our species and condition will be manifested in any one life. The rest will be held in abeyance until we reincarnate into another species where the conditions are appropriate to them.

♦ We have deep impressions of our past thoughts and actions and these will remain as memories, whether conscious or unconscious. Even if we evolve into another species in a different time, our karma will still continue to operate.

♦ Since the desire to live is eternal, our tendencies and past impressions are beginning-less.

♦ Karma only operates and produces behavioural patterns for as long as we have certain obstacles: ignorance, attachment, egoism, aversion, and the desire to cling to life. When we remove these obstacles, we remove the karma.

♦ The past is present with us through the emotions and feelings that once arose; the future is present with us through our hopes and expectations. How they manifest depend on our circumstances, as well as individual and universal laws.

♦ The three forces of Nature – dark and heavy inertia, speedy activity and light, transparent clarity – govern when and how these individual and universal laws affect us.

♦ Since these three forces of Nature work together within every change of form and expression, there is a unity in all things.

23. The Mind, the World and the Self

♦ Since we all have different minds, we all see the same object differently. Therefore the mind must be other than the object.

♦ The object exists independently whether the mind

perceives it or not. If that were not the case, what would happen to that object when the mind was not perceiving it?

- ♦ The mind perceives objects or ignores them depending on whether we are attracted to or interested in the object.
- ♦ Although the Self, the ruler of the mind, does not change, it knows and is the master of the mind's fluctuations.
- ♦ The mind is not self-luminous since it is also an object of perception.
- ♦ The mind can, as a subject, perceive external objects. It can also turn within and reflect the Self, so it can be either subject or object.
- ♦ If we had two minds, one an object of knowledge and the second the subjective knower, there would be even greater confusion. The second mind would perceive the first, the mind would become aware of itself and there would be an endless proliferation of sources of consciousness.
- ♦ The pure awareness of the Self is unchangeable. When the mind is not turned outward, it reflects this pure awareness itself. We must understand the external origin of our thoughts so that we can discover the state where our mind reflects awareness rather than objects.
- ♦ The mind is able to perceive because it reflects both the Self and the objects of perception, allowing it to understand everything.
- ♦ Although the mind has many desires and impressions, it can only exist for the sake of the Self, because it can only act in association with the Self.
- ♦ When we understand the difference between the mind and the Self, we no longer assume that the thoughts in our mind come from the Self.

24. Liberated Consciousness

◆ When our mind moves towards discernment, spontaneously making the right choices at the right time, we approach a state of serenity and liberation.

◆ If our mind relaxes and stops discriminating, then distracting thoughts will arise, because of our past impressions and conditioning.

◆ These past impressions can be removed as we have previously seen.

◆ When we possess all the psychic powers and can remain totally disinterested even in the highest rewards of meditation, our discernment and perfect discrimination take us to the state of samadhi known as the 'cloud of virtue'.

◆ Then our ignorance ceases, we no longer have any suffering and we are free from the power of karma.

◆ Then all the impurities of knowledge are gone, and the universe no longer holds any secrets; we know the nature of everything in the universe.

◆ Then the three forces of Nature stop their sequence of transformation because they have fulfilled their purpose.

◆ For the illumined Self, time has no reality. There is no sequence in thought patterns, and He controls time, knowing the past, present and future as a moment in the eternal now.

◆ The Self is realized. It achieves its purpose by being established in its own pure awareness. You just rest in your own true nature.

Glory unto those who have realized their own nature.
May you attain purity of heart in your lives.